MW01165373

Peripherally Inserted Central Venous Catheters

Sergio Sandrucci • Baudolino Mussa
Editors

Peripherally Inserted Central Venous Catheters

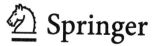 Springer

Editors

Sergio Sandrucci
Visceral Sarcoma and Rare Cancers Unit
University of Turin Medical School
Turin
Italy

Baudolino Mussa
Digestive, Colorectal and Oncological
Surgery Unit
University of Turin Medical School
Turin
Italy

ISBN 978-88-470-5664-0   ISBN 978-88-470-5665-7   (eBook)
DOI 10.1007/978-88-470-5665-7
Springer Milan Heidelberg New York Dordrecht London

Library of Congress Control Number: 2014941895

© Springer-Verlag Italia 2014
This work is subject to copyright. All rights are reserved by the Publisher, whether the whole or part of the material is concerned, specifically the rights of translation, reprinting, reuse of illustrations, recitation, broadcasting, reproduction on microfilms or in any other physical way, and transmission or information storage and retrieval, electronic adaptation, computer software, or by similar or dissimilar methodology now known or hereafter developed. Exempted from this legal reservation are brief excerpts in connection with reviews or scholarly analysis or material supplied specifically for the purpose of being entered and executed on a computer system, for exclusive use by the purchaser of the work. Duplication of this publication or parts thereof is permitted only under the provisions of the Copyright Law of the Publisher's location, in its current version, and permission for use must always be obtained from Springer. Permissions for use may be obtained through RightsLink at the Copyright Clearance Center. Violations are liable to prosecution under the respective Copyright Law.
The use of general descriptive names, registered names, trademarks, service marks, etc. in this publication does not imply, even in the absence of a specific statement, that such names are exempt from the relevant protective laws and regulations and therefore free for general use.
While the advice and information in this book are believed to be true and accurate at the date of publication, neither the authors nor the editors nor the publisher can accept any legal responsibility for any errors or omissions that may be made. The publisher makes no warranty, express or implied, with respect to the material contained herein.

Printed on acid-free paper

Springer is part of Springer Science+Business Media (www.springer.com)

Preface

Peripherally inserted central catheters (PICCs), used since the 1940s for hemodynamic measurement and with a limited clinical role, were reintroduced in the 1970s as an alternative to non-tunnelled central vascular catheters (CVCs) for the delivery of total parenteral nutrition. Initially, polyethylene catheters were used, but their use was hampered by high complication rates, specifically thrombophlebitis and catheter sepsis.

With advances in materials design and the use of echography to guide catheter insertion, the use of PICCs has gained wider application in home-based IV therapies as well. In both clinical and home-health settings, PICCs have been shown to adequately and safely meet the needs of patients under short- or long-term therapy. The spread of ultrasound guidance as gold standard for positioning has radically changed the history of vascular access in terms of eliminating complications and improving the success rates of the manoeuvre. Since the beginning of this century, virtually all PICCs are inserted by this technique and the results of insertions have dramatically changed.

The ultrasound guidance allows the cannulation of the arm's deep veins (especially basilica and brachial veins), using a modified Seldinger technique which allows to obtain an extremely low failure rate as well as very few potential complications at the time of insertion. Above all, the exit site is located in an area defined by some American authors the "green zone", in the middle of the arm, midway between the elbow and armpit, with low bacterial colonization and perfect for a stable and lasting medication.

PICCs have the great virtue of having promoted the great revolution in facing venous access issues through a team approach, opening new and exiting perspectives in nursing and management thanks to the concept of "PICC team". A team is defined as a group of individuals with a set of complementary skills required to complete a task, job, or project: team members are accountable for collective performance and work towards common goals with shared rewards. A PICC team is not likely to be built in an institution through having nurses trained to place PICC lines in their spare time. Moreover, PICC teams do not necessarily work towards a common goal in synergy. A PICC team is likely to have multiple members and may perform multiple tasks that include care and maintenance as well as troubleshooting and clinical staff education.

Concerning this aspect, the availability of a reliable approach to central venous system opens the way to the so-called proactive approach. In the long term, the use of a proactive assessment of the patient's vascular access needs (based on the type of therapy the patient will be receiving, included the length of therapy, drug characteristics, vessel health and any comorbidities the patient may be dealing with) helps to protect patient's vascular integrity while providing safe and cost-effective vascular access.

The proactive approach to vessel health and preservation requires a multidisciplinary team evaluation of the patient's vasculature and the planned therapy. While somewhat challenging to implement, this approach results in vessel preservation, on-time therapy, and improved patient outcomes.

For all of these reasons our belief is that a practical state-of-the-art guide dealing with the different issues concerning PICC choice, positioning and management is extremely useful.

This book was conceived to face the topic of PICC starting from an overview of the history of venous accesses, going on with the ultrasound anatomy of peripheral veins and ultrasound guided venipuncture maneuvers, precautions and tricks focused to PICC positioning procedure; clinical problems associated to the use of peripheral venous approaches in clinical practice (including infections and thrombosis) are also faced. Ethical, psychological and legal aspects concerning peripherally inserted central catheters, and off-label use of these devices are also discussed.

The editors are very grateful to the many experts and colleagues that cooperated with us with tremendous experience and skill and, of course, availability. We sincerely thank all these colleagues for their highly valued support.

Turin, Italy   Sergio Sandrucci
February 2014   Baudolino Mussa

Contents

Introduction and Overview of PICC History

Roberto Biffi

Although peripheral IV (intravenous) cannulation is the most common means for administration of routine infusions, the risk of infiltration, accidental dislodgements, need for frequent replacement, and thrombotic complication render IV cannulation of peripheral veins with short catheters inadequate for circumstances in which long-term or central access is desired. Parenteral nutrition (PN) and chronic hemodialysis – both in the hospital and the outpatient setting – are historically the first, most common, and lifesaving methods of therapy made possible by modern technical advances in achieving and maintaining safe vascular access.

Before the seventeenth century, scientists and physicians did not understand the physiology of blood vessels and body fluids, until *Harvey* introduced them to the concepts of experimentation and biologic research. Nevertheless, the Egyptians in the Edwin Smith and Ebers papyri (circa 1550 BC) described 22 blood vessels which carried air, liquids, and waste materials and were connected to the heart, and the Romans had precision tools, which can be clearly identified in a surgeon's house in Pompeii devastated by the eruption of Vesuvius in AD 67. Harvey first described the *circulatory system* in 1616; he discovered that the heart circulates the blood throughout the body, acting as both a muscle and a pump and producing a continuous circulation of the blood. Until that time, it was believed that, although arteries and veins contained blood, the blood flowed like *human breath*. Indeed, until Harvey subsequently identified the capillary network, the liver was regarded as the center of the circulatory system. Well into the nineteenth century, many physicians believed that a *useless abundance of blood* was a principal cause of all disease, and accordingly, blood was commonly removed with lancets, cupping, and leeches. Bloodletting was a common practice in the past, and venesection was performed by specialists for the treatment of fevers and apoplexy. Hippocrates describes the best method of

R. Biffi
Department of Abdomino-Pelvic and Minimally Invasive Surgery,
European Institute of Oncology, Via Ripamonti 435, Milan 20141, Italy
e-mail: roberto.biffi@ieo.it

S. Sandrucci, B. Mussa (eds.), *Peripherally Inserted Central Venous Catheters,*
DOI 10.1007/978-88-470-5665-7_1, © Springer-Verlag Italia 2014

venesection in his book Regimen in Acute Diseases: "… if the vein is to be cut, do so at the elbow and draw plenty of blood."

After the pioneering activity of Harvey, in February 1665, Dr Richard Lower demonstrated a successful blood transfusion from a cervical artery of one dog to a jugular vein of another. Previous vein-to-vein experiments had been unsuccessful because of the clotting of the slow movement of the venous blood. In 1877, Nikolai Vladimirovich Eck reported his experience with the creation of a fistula between the canine portal vein and inferior vena cava using a continuous silk suture. This was probably the first direct vascular anastomosis. Vascular anastomoses were then performed in Europe by Jassinowsky in 1889 and Jaboulay in 1896. *Alexis Carrel* in association with Charles G. Guthrie was the most acknowledged for early vascular surgery. Carrel was presented with a Nobel Prize in 1912 for a work published in 1902 dealing with technical aspects of vascular anastomoses.

In 1966, Brescia et al. [1] reported the creation of an *arteriovenous fistula* in the forearm to ensure a venous blood flow of 250–300 mL per minute. They had found cannula morbidity, revisions, and clotting were a frequent cause of hospitalization of dialysis patients. Single-needle dialysis, described by Kopp in 1972, has been replaced by double-lumen needle dialysis because of superior blood flow and clearance characteristics. In most cases, *hemodialysis* by catheter is reserved for acute and short-term use, particularly during the period of maturation of an internal fistula.

The pivotal development in providing opportunity for successful long-term infusion of hypertonic PN solutions was the accomplishment of consistently safe and effective central venous access by percutaneous infraclavicular *subclavian vein catheterization*. Although methods for gaining vascular access have been evolving and have been recorded for three and a half centuries (and likely were attempted even much earlier), practical central venous access is a relatively recent achievement of the past 60 years (Table 1.1). The primary development in the most frequently used route of central venous access today was the first successful percutaneous catheterization of the subclavian vein for blood transfusion in critically wounded French military personnel in 1952 by Aubaniac [2]. Within the next two years, this novel technique was subsequently used and developed further as a means of emergency central venous access for rapid volume resuscitation. The supraclavicular approach to percutaneous subclavian vein catheterization as a means of access for rapid fluid resuscitation was first described a few years later by Yoffa in 1965. During this time period, various percutaneous external and internal jugular vein catheter insertion techniques had also been used for venous access for fluid resuscitation in adults and for transfusion in infants before being used by Dudrick et al. [3] and Wilmore and Dudrick [4] as the initial route of central venous access for infusion of PN solutions both in adults and infants.

The first plastic (polyethylene) catheter for IV infusion was inserted into a vein either as a cutdown or by passing it through the lumen of a needle percutaneously in 1950 at Mayo Clinic by an anesthesiology resident [5]. As a consequence, rubber tubing was replaced by plastic tubing for routine IV administration.

Table 1.1 Highlights in the development of venous access

1616	
First description of the circulation in *Excercitatio Anatomica de Moto Cordis et Sanguinis in Animalibus*. *Harvey*	
1665	
Transfusion of blood from one live dog to another using quills to transfer blood from a carotid artery of the donor to a jugular vein of the recipient. *Lower*	
1818	
First successful blood transfusion into a woman dying of severe postpartum hemorrhage with blood obtained from a man using 8-oz syringes. *Blundell*	
1831	
IV infusion of water and saline for successful treatment of cholera in human beings *O'Shaughnessy, Latta*	
1877	
First creation of a fistula between the canine portal vein and inferior vena cava using a continuous silk suture. This was probably the first direct vascular anastomosis. *Eck*	
1912	
Carrel presented with a Nobel Prize for a work published in 1902 dealing with technical aspects of vascular anastomoses. *Carrel*	
1945	
First polyethylene plastic catheter for IV infusion introduced into a vein by passing it through the lumen of a needle. Later developed and made available commercially as Intracath (BD Worldwide, Franklin Lakes, NJ). *Zimmermann*	
1950	
Development of the Rochester plastic needle by an anesthesiology resident at the Mayo Clinic. Rubber tubing replaced by plastic tubing for routine IV administration. *Massa*	
1952	
First description of subclavian percutaneous venipuncture to achieve rapid transfusion in severely injured war victims. *Aubaniac*	
1952	
First description of the technique of inserting and advancing catheters for interventional radiology over a flexible J-wire inserted into an artery or vein through a needle. *Seldinger*	
1960	
Central venous catheters inserted peripherally in upper and lower extremity veins for monitoring central venous pressure primarily in cardiac surgery patients and critically ill patients. *Wilson*	
1966	
Creation of an arteriovenous fistula in the forearm to assure a venous blood flow of 250–300 mL per minute. *Brescia, Cimino, Appel, Hunvich*	
1966	
Central venous polyvinyl catheters inserted into superior vena cava of beagle puppies via jugular veins. Puppies grew and developed normally. *Dudrick, Vars, Rhoads*	
1967	
First comprehensive technique for long-term parenteral nutrition (PN) via central venous catheters inserted by percutaneous puncture of an external jugular or internal jugular vein. *Dudrick*	
1973	
Silicone rubber catheter with attached Dacron cuff (for fixation by ingrowth of tissue) developed for insertion into superior vena cava for infusion and tunneled subcutaneously to exit on the chest. *Broviac, Cole, Scribner*	

(continued)

Table 1.1 (continued)

1975
Introduction of first peripherally inserted central venous silicone catheter. *Hoshal*
1979
Broviac catheter modified by increasing wall thickness and lumen diameter. Double-lumen silicone rubber Dacron-cuffed catheter developed for ambulatory home PN and chemotherapy. Triple-lumen version was also designed to allow blood sampling in addition to infusions. *Hickman, Buckner, Clift, Sanders, Stewart, Thomas*
1982
Introduction of implantable infusion chambers (ports or TIAP) or chronic venous access devices (CVAD), placed surgically in subcutaneous pockets
Specially ground needles (Huber) designed to prevent coring of the entry site, intermittently placed through a self-sealing silicone rubber diaphragm after appropriate antimicrobial skin preparation. *Niederhuber, Ensminger, Gyves, Liepman, Doan, Cozzi*
1984
Percutaneous translumbar and transhepatic inferior vena caval catheters inserted for prolonged vascular access for both inpatient and ambulatory home PN. *Dudrick, O'Donnell, Englert*
2007–2009
Introduction of Power ports and Power PICCs, proposed for their ability to withstand the pressure created by power contrast media injectors during contrast-enhanced computed tomography. *Some international manufacturing companies*

The decision to abandon peripheral venous infusion in favor of central venous infusion as the preferred route for providing all required nutrients entirely by vein was a key factor leading to the successful development and clinical application of PN. The quantity of high-quality nutrients required to achieve and maintain positive nitrogen balance and its associated clinical benefits in a critically ill patient had to be concentrated in a volume of water that could be tolerated without untoward complications. The resulting hypertonic nutrient solutions exceeded the *normal osmolarity* of the circulating blood approximately sixfold (1,800 mOsm/L) or more. The infusion of hypertonic solutions of this magnitude into peripheral veins caused an intolerable degree of pain, together with an inevitable and unjustifiable inflammation of the intima of the vein and damage to the formed elements of the blood, resulting in inordinate phlebitis and *thrombophlebitis* and associated adverse secondary consequences and complications. However, it was discovered and demonstrated in the animal laboratory, and subsequently confirmed in human subjects and patients, that hypertonic solutions, when infused at a constant rate over the 24 h of each day through a catheter with its tip in a large central vein, such as the superior vena cava, were rapidly diluted virtually to iso-osmolarity by the high blood flow (50 % of cardiac output) in this major vein.

In 1979, the Hickman catheter, a long-term venous access device, was used for chemotherapy for the first time [6]. The introduction of totally implantable vascular access devices (TIVAD) started in the early 1980s [7].

Prior to the development of polyurethane and silicone catheters, central venous polyethylene or polyvinyl catheters placed in the upper arm by passing them through the lumen of a needle percutaneously, accessing superficial, visible veins of the forearm or the elbow, were not well tolerated, and thrombophlebitis almost always occurred within a few days after implantation of these devices.

Production of novel and better-tolerated materials allowed for the introduction of modern PICCs (peripherally inserted central catheters) in the mid-1970s [8]. A modern PICC is a 50–60-cm-long vascular access device with entry into the basilic, cephalic, or brachial veins of the middle to upper arm. Although a PICC is inserted peripherally, the tip resides in a central position (the distal superior vena cava or atrio-caval junction). Whereas midline catheters (IV catheter whose tip terminates in a vein in the upper arm and not in a central location) and peripheral IV cannulae are restricted to infusions of medications and fluids between a pH of 5 and 9 and can tolerate an osmolarity up to 500–600 mOsm/L, PICCs can essentially be used for any infusion, regardless of pH and osmolarity, and can protect the veins from medications and fluids that are irritants or vesicants, such as chemotherapeutic agents and parenteral nutrition.

A great improvement was the adoption of *micro-introducer technique* in the 1980s, as the traditional method for PICC insertion was vein access using a peel-away introducer often as large as 14 gauge and many factors negatively impacted the success of such an approach. The veins might be too small, scarred from previous therapies, or the patient might experience venous spasm. Successful placement using this conventional approach was at that time reported to be as low as 55 % to as high as 70 %, and patients with poor veins had to be often referred to interventional radiologists for catheter placement without a bedside attempt.

Placement of PICCs using systematically the micro-introducer technique (*modified Seldinger technique* or MST) became in the 1980s the standard of practice, due to the increased success of placement over the traditional method of peel-away introducer. Placement of PICCs using MST improved the practitioner's ability to access veins above the antecubital fossa, paired with *ultrasound guidance*. Vascular ultrasound uses a probe that sends high-frequency waves through the tissue: the size, vein condition, location, and arteries can be identified. Ultrasound is used to guide a small-gauge needle into veins that may not be palpable or visible to the naked eye. When MST and ultrasound are used concurrently, successful insertion is now reported in the range of 92–100 %, with reduced complications and patients' costs for PICC maintenance [9].

Patients requiring long-term medications over weeks to months, or even short-term infusions of caustic medications or fluids, should be considered for PICC placement. Placing a PICC allows for the administration of an entire range of infusates including parenteral nutrition, chemotherapy, antibiotics, blood components, IV fluids for hydration, and incompatible drugs. PICCs may also be used for blood sampling; patients in need of frequent venipuncture for blood sampling may benefit from a PICC because blood draws could cause anxiety and dissatisfaction. Although most manufacturers do not recommend sampling blood from catheters smaller than 3.8F to 4F because of the risk of catheter occlusion, studies have shown that blood can be safely drawn from catheters as small as 3F, the most commonly used PICC size in pediatric patients.

Peripherally inserted central catheter survival times and rates of therapy completion with a single catheter vary across indications and studies. Proper indication and correct nursing allow for long-term performance of these devices, up to years in some well-managed cases. In a long-term study – carried out in pediatric cancer patients in India – elective removal occurred in 63/101 (62.4 %) PICCs and removal due to complications resulted in a complication rate of 2.41 per 1,000 catheter days [10]. Usual *rates of completion of therapy* with a single PICC range from 62% to 82 %, with higher completion rates among outpatient populations and patients requiring shorter courses of parenteral therapy.

By the 1990s, 85 % of hospitalized patients received IV therapy at some point in their hospitalization, and the practice of IV therapy expanded to physicians' offices and other outpatient services while developing into a major home care modality. Over the last few decades, many management changes in oncology have occurred, particularly with respect to new chemotherapy combinations and more complex application schemes. Cancer patients usually require repeated venous punctures for treatment monitoring, application of chemotherapy, or blood transfusions. According to recent US data, approximately 150 million intravenous catheters are purchased and at least 5 million central venous catheters are inserted every year. Recently, marketed PICCs may have a single, double, or triple lumen, usually with an outer diameter of between two and seven French gauge. Some newer catheters are now proposed for their ability to also provide for monitoring of central venous pressure and to withstand the pressure created by power contrast media injectors during diagnostic procedures (*Power ports* and *Power PICCs*), thus allowing the use of these devices in many clinical conditions, ranging from prolonged chemotherapy to intensive care. Technological advancements in the future will inevitably produce devices which will be even safer, more reliable, and more cost-effective.

References

1. Brescia MJ, Cimino JE, Appel K, Hunvich BJ (1966) Chronic hemodialysis using venipuncture and a surgically created arteriovenous fistula. N Engl J Med 275:1089–1092
2. Aubaniac R (1952) Subclavian intravenous injection: advantages and technic. Presse Med 60:1456
3. Dudrick SJ, Wilmore DW, Vars HM, Rhoads JE (1968) Long-term total parenteral nutrition with growth, development, and positive nitrogen balance. Surgery 64:134–142
4. Wilmore DW, Dudrick SJ (1968) Growth and development of an infant receiving all nutrients exclusively by vein. JAMA 203:860–864
5. Massa DJ, Lundy JS, Faulconer A Jr, Ridley RW (1950) A plastic needle. Proc Staff Meet Mayo Clin 25:413–415
6. Hickman RO, Buckner CD, Clift RA et al (1979) A modified right atrial catheter for access to the venous system in marrow transplant recipients. Surg Gynecol Obstet 148:871–875
7. Niederhuber JE, Ensminger W, Gyves JW et al (1982) Totally implanted venous and arterial access system to replace external catheters in cancer treatment. Surgery 92:706–712
8. Hoshal VL (1975) Total intravenous nutrition with peripherally inserted silicone elastomer central venous catheters. Arch Surg 110:644–646
9. Li J, Fan YY, Xin MZ et al (2013) A randomised, controlled trial comparing the long-term effects of peripherally inserted central catheter placement in chemotherapy patients using B-mode ultrasound with modified Seldinger technique versus blind puncture. Eur J Oncol Nurs 2014;18(1):94–103
10. Abedin S, Kapoor G (2008) Peripherally inserted central venous catheters are a good option for prolonged venous access in children with cancer. Pediatr Blood Cancer 51:251–255

Which Material and Device?
The Choice of PICC

2

Enrico de Lutio

2.1 Introduction

Until a few years ago, the medium- to long-term central venous catheters (CVC) were essentially silicone (SR) catheters. Silicone was the material of choice for the vascular access devices (VADs) including PICCs.

Nowadays, the newest polyurethanes (PUR) are available, and their features increase therapy options accomplishable with these devices with indubitable advantages for patient's outcome.

It is fair to say that there are no data from clinical studies that prove the superiority of one of those two materials in all the situations, but there are circumstances in which it makes sense to choose one of the materials for its superiority with regard to particular aspects.

So, therefore, the clinical implications of material properties can certainly influence vascular access device (VAD) selection with regard to ease of insertion, mechanical phlebitis, flow rates, infusate compatibility, extravasation of infusates, catheter occlusion, clotting and thrombosis, catheter weakening and embolization, vascular damage, stability and durability, and catheter maintenance requirements.

2.2 PICC Structure and Materials

Every venous catheter is made up of two parts: the intravascular part and the extravascular one.

The intravascular segment is usually made of one of the two abovementioned materials, while the extravascular segment can have different materials due to the several components like clamps and the hub.

E. de Lutio
Consultant, Via P. Carleni, 2, Amelia (TR) 05022, Italy
e-mail: enrico.delutio@googlemail.com

S. Sandrucci, B. Mussa (eds.), *Peripherally Inserted Central Venous Catheters*,
DOI 10.1007/978-88-470-5665-7_2, © Springer-Verlag Italia 2014

Table 2.1 Materials

Family	Polimer	Acronyme
Polyolefin	Polyethylene	PE
	Polypropylene	PP
Vynilic	Polyvinyl chloride and derivates	PVCPS ABS
Styrenic	Polystyrene	PS
	Poly (acrylonitrile-butadiene-styrene)	ABS
Acrylics	Poly (methyl-methacrylate)	PMMA
Polyamides	Polyamide	PA
Polyesters saturated	Polyethylene terephthalate	PET
Polycarbonate	Polycarbonates	PC
Polyacetals	Polyoxymethylene	POM
Fluoroelastomers	Polytetrafluoroethylene	PTFE
	Polyvinylidene fluoride	PVDF
Silicon	Silicon	SIL
Polyurethanes	Polyurethanes aromatic and aliphatic	PUR

The knowledge of the material of such components is important because it can be damaged by the liquids used for skin disinfection, for the scrubbing of the needle-less valved connectors, etc.

There is a huge variety of materials (Table 2.1) that must be taken into right consideration.

2.3   Silicone (SR)

Silicone materials have been used in medicine for almost six decades. Available in a variety of material types, they have unique chemical and physical properties that manifest in excellent biocompatibility and biodurability for many applications [1].

Their high biocompatibility is explained with their remarkable chemical stability that enables biocompatibility in many long-term implant applications.

Silicones are a general category of synthetic polymers whose backbone is made of repeating silicon to oxygen bonds. In addition to their links to oxygen to form the polymeric chain, the silicone atoms are also bonded to organic groups, typically methyl groups. This is the basis for the name "silicones," which was assigned by Kipping based on their similarity with ketones, because in most cases, there is on average one silicone atom for one oxygen and two methyl groups [2]. Later, as these materials and their applications flourished, more specific nomenclature was developed. The basic repeating unit became known as "siloxane," and the most common silicone is polydimethylsiloxane, abbreviated as PMDS (Fig. 2.1):

Polysiloxanes are polymers made up of a chain of small repeating units with an end group. They tend to be chemically inert due to the strength of the silicon-oxygen bond.

Fig. 2.1 Silicone and PUR formulation

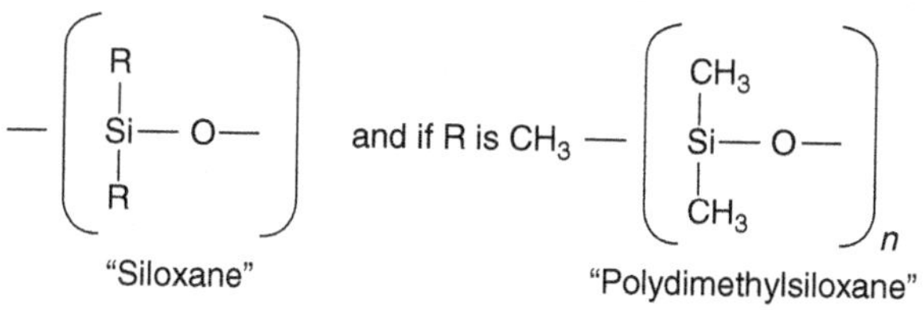

Furthermore, surface-active additives can be mixed with the polymer, or added to the ends of the polymer chain, to modify its surface properties [3].

For medical applications, the silicone must be medical grade. Medical-grade silicone has special requirements that are different from industrial-grade silicone. The major difference is that the silicone manufacturers have a special silicone grade that they manufacture for medical application. These silicones are tested for biocompatibility and meet the necessary regulatory body requirements. Any additives such as color must also be medical grade. Medical silicone applications are divided into two classes: restricted and unrestricted. Normally, restricted is referred to as short-term implantable and unrestricted is referred to as long-term implantable.

2.4 Polyurethane (PUR)

Otto (Friedrich) Bayer (1902–1982) and coworkers discovered and patented the chemistry of polyurethanes in 1937, and the first true medical-grade elastomeric polyurethanes were patented in 1960 by du Pont (Pierce et al.) called Biomer® (trade name Lycra) [3].

Today, polyurethanes (PURs) are a class of polymer, which has achieved industrial relevance due to their rough and elastomeric properties and good fatigue resistance and has been employed in biomaterial applications such as artificial pacemaker lead insulation, catheters, and vascular grafts [1].

Polyurethanes consist of a class of materials with widely varying physical and chemical properties.

The commonality is the urethane linkage between polymer chains made up of isocyanate (hard segment, aromatic, or aliphatic), macroglycol (soft segment, polyesters; polyethers or polycarbonates), and chain extender (diols; diamines) (Fig. 2.2).

The hard segments are glassy or crystalline with the use of temperature, while the other segment – the soft segment – is rubbery.

Polyurethane hard segments consist of either aliphatic (carbon polymer backbones with single bonds between Cs) or aromatic (backbones with single and double bonds) di-isocyanates.

The isocyanate monomers are toxic, and their removal is essential for use in PURs for biomedical applications.

With regard to soft segments, for catheter applications, polyether and polycarbonate soft segments are used.

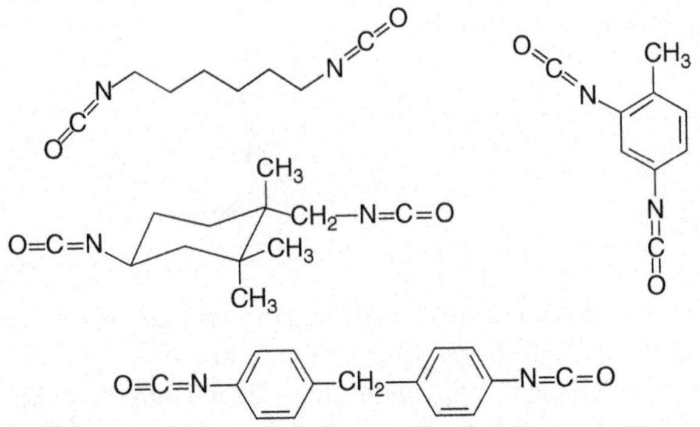

Fig. 2.2 Uretahne linkage

Table 2.2 PUR brand names

Brand name	Chemical composition
Tecoflex	Aliphatic polyether
Tecothane	Aromatic polyether
Carbothane	Aliphatic polycarbonate
Chronoflex	Aliphatic polycarbonate
Pellethane	Aromatic polyether

PURs with polycarbonate soft segments are more resistant to attack by biological enzymes and hydrolysis than those made with polyethers.

Polyurethane properties are notoriously difficult to control because of the number of components in the polymer and the requirement for tight control of polymerization conditions.

Some catheter manufacturers require prefiltering of all components to assure purity of monomers.

The final polymer is also filtered to assure a consistent molecular weight and tight molecular weight distribution.

Each lot is individually inspected to assure conformance with specifications and is only released after review of all documentation.

PUR materials are varied by altering the composition of the hard and soft segments, as well as the length of the segment chains.

The processing of the polymer also plays a role in determining the properties of the finished catheter.

Examples of commercially available PUs used in medical applications are in the Table 2.2.

2.5   SR vs. PUR Catheter Material Properties

Once showed the physical and chemical differences between silicones and PUs, we can now see what such differences implicate in terms of functions of all CVCs including PICCs.

2 Which Material and Device? The Choice of PICC

11

First of all, let us look at the physical tests and material properties which are used to evaluate and describe the strength and resilience of catheter tubing to certain environmental conditions [3].

Some of the most common of these are:

- Tensile strength
- Burst strength
- Flow rates
- Kink resistance
- Durometer (hardness)
- Flexural modulus (stiffness)
- Environmental stress cracking
- Solvent resistance
- Drug compatibility

2.5.1 Tensile Strength

The ultimate tensile strength (UTS), often shortened to tensile strength (TS) or ultimate strength, is the maximum stress that a material can withstand while being stretched or pulled before failing or breaking [1, 2, 4, 5].

In the case of catheters, a measure of the maximum force that can be applied to the catheter before it breaks.

Silicone catheters have much less tensile strength than polyurethane catheters with identical dimensions.

2.5.2 Burst Strength

Pressure at which a film or sheet (e.g., of paper or plastic) will burst. Used as a measure of resistance to rupture, burst strength depends largely on the tensile strength and extensibility of the material.

In the case of catheters, the burst strength is the pressure applied to a catheter lumen of a closed catheter that causes it to leak.

Silicone catheters have lower burst strength than polyurethane catheters with identical dimensions.

2.5.3 Flow Rates

Because SR has lower tensile and burst strength than PUR catheters of equal dimensions, the wall thickness of SR catheters is increased to provide adequate strength.

Consequently, for the same catheter French size, SR catheters have a smaller lumen and lower flow rate than PUR catheters.

Flow is proportional to r4, so very small changes in inside diameter dimension – especially of small-diameter catheters – have a very large effect on flow rates.

2.5.4   Kink Resistance

Kink resistance is the ability of the catheter to maintain an open lumen when bent.

SR catheters bend more easily than polyurethane and, in general, can be bent to larger angles before kinking but kink with less applied force than PUR catheters. SR catheters also recover more readily or are not permanently deformed as easily as are PUR catheters.

2.5.5   Durometer (Hardness)

Durometer is one of several measures of the hardness of a material.

Hardness may be defined as a material's resistance to permanent indentation. The durometer scale was defined by Albert F. Shore, who developed a measurement device called a durometer in the 1920s. The term durometer is often used to refer to the measurement, as well as the instrument itself. Durometer is typically used as a measure of hardness in polymers, elastomers, and rubbers.

Useful because it is easily determined and reflects "catheter feel" – i.e., whether it is soft and pliable or stiff.

SR catheters, in general, are made of materials with lower durometer than

PUR catheters and are, therefore, floppier, even though they have greater wall thickness.

2.5.6   Flexural Modulus (Stiffness)

A measure of the ease with which a catheter can be bent.

SR materials have lower flexural moduli than PUR materials, and consequently SR catheters are usually less stiff.

The easiest way to compare is to let equal lengths of catheters extend over a table and see which one bends more under the force of gravity.

2.5.7   Environmental Stress Cracking

When subject to repeated cycles of chemical and mechanical stress, cracks can form in the surface of a material and grow into the bulk, eventually leading to failure.

SR is less prone to stress cracking than PUR because it is cross-linked and is also more resistant to attack by common antiseptic and cleaning preparations (Fig. 2.3).

2.5.8   Solvent Resistance

Solvent resistance is a measure of the ability of a material to retain its properties when exposed to chemicals.

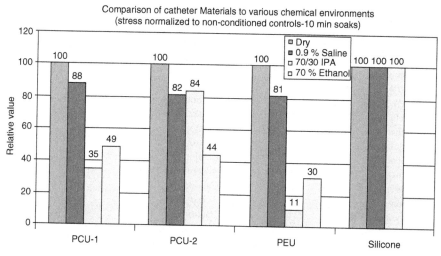

Fig. 2.3 Materials and their resistance to various chemical environments

SR is more resistant to solvents in general, because it is cross-linked. SR catheters swell, but do not break in most solvents. SR's hydrophobicity limits its attack by water.

2.5.9 Drug Compatibility

It is important to know that catheters are not attacked by drugs, but by the solvents necessary to put them into solution or to preserve them [3]. Therefore, drug compatibility is based upon the solvent or carrier compatibility with the polymer.

Drugs diffuse through SR catheters to a lesser extent than most PUR catheters (dependent on chemical composition and structure of the PUR), because drugs can only diffuse while in solution (Table 2.3).

2.5.10 Radiopacity

Radiopacity is a function of the amount of radiopaque material in the fluoroscopic image of the catheter. Smaller-diameter catheters or catheters loaded with a lower concentration of radiopaque agent have less presence and present therefore appear dimmer.

Radiopacity is achieved thanks to the addition of radiopaque agents (i.e., $BaSO_4$) to the SR or PUR, but they weaken catheter materials by increasing their rigidity.

Imaging of thicker-walled catheters is better than that of thinner-walled catheters if loading is the same.

Table 2.3 Chemicals and their impact on PUR

Chemical	Impact on PU
Taxol	Caution
Taxotere	Caution
.9 % saline	Acceptable
4–5 % IPA	Acceptable
70 % IPA	Caution
4–5 % ethanol	Acceptable
70 % ethanol	Caution
TPA solutions (i.e. Lyposin)	Caution
Polysorbate 80	Caution
Hibiciens (4 % IPA)	Acceptable
Chloraprep (70 % IPA)	Caution
3 % hydrogen peroxide	Acceptable
Povidone iodine solution	Caution
Betadine ointment	Caution
Acetone	Caution

2.5.11 Biocompatibility

Biocompatibility is related to the behavior of biomaterials in various contexts.

There are several definitions of "biocompatibility":

"The ability of a material to perform with an appropriate host response in a specific application," Williams' definition or "The quality of not having toxic or injurious effects on biological systems" [6, 7].

"Comparison of the tissue response produced through the close association of the implanted candidate material to its implant site within the host animal to that tissue response recognized and established as suitable with control materials." ASTM (American Society for Testing and Materials)

"Refers to the ability of a biomaterial to perform its desired function with respect to a medical therapy, without eliciting any undesirable local or systemic effects in the recipient or beneficiary of that therapy, but generating the most appropriate beneficial cellular or tissue response in that specific situation, and optimizing the clinically relevant performance of that therapy" [8].

"Biocompatibility is the capability of a prosthesis implanted in the body to exist in harmony with tissue without causing deleterious changes".

With regard to venous catheters, the main biological issue for catheters is hemocompatibility and, to a lesser extent, compatibility with tissue contacted to access the vessel lumen.

Hemocompatibility is a complex issue. Depending on how it is defined, on the patient population, disease state, catheter entrance site, and other factors (phase of the moon?), one catheter material can be said to perform better, or worse, than another.

For short-term applications, in general, there are no noticeable differences between PUR and SR catheters.

For longer-term applications, durability may be more important than biocompatibility.

Table 2.4 Differences between materials and properties

Property	Silicone	Polyurethane
Strength (tensile, burst, tear)	Poor, fair	Good, excellent
Placement stiffness	Fair	Good, excellent
In-situ stiffness	Excellent	Excellent
Bend radius	Excellent radius	Fair, good, excellent
Kink resistance	Fair, good kink	Excellent kink
Implant stability	Excellent	Good, excellent
Chemical resistance	Excellent	Fair, good
Size/flow ratio	Fair	Excellent
Availability	Excellent	Excellent
Biocompatibility	Excellent	Excellent

Once the differences between silicone and polyurethanes in terms of material properties are seen, let us take a look at the following figure that recaps those differences (Table 2.4).

2.6   Clinical Implications of Material Properties That Influence Catheter Selection

For the ultimate purpose of this book, the simple listing of the properties of the SR vs. PUR catheter material would be pretty useless if those properties were not associated with their clinical implications, assessed in terms of:
- Ease of insertion
- Mechanical phlebitis
- Flow rates
- Infusate compatibility
- Extravasation of infusates
- Catheter occlusion
- Clotting and thrombosis
- Catheter weakening and embolization
- Vascular damage
- Stability/durability
- Catheter maintenance requirements

2.6.1   Ease of Insertion

The ease of insertion is influenced by catheter stiffness, wall thickness, and frictional properties of catheter surface.

In general, SR catheters are more difficult to advance over the guidewire than PUR catheters of same dimensions because they have higher surface friction to the guidewire.

For other catheters than venous accesses or PICCs, it can be compensated for by applying hydrophilic coating on the guidewire or jacketing guidewires in Teflon®.

The PICCs are inserted with the modified Seldinger technique in which the guidewire is only used for a few centimeters and just for the introduction of the Peel-Away introducer and therefore the abovementioned possible issues are not a concern.

2.6.2   Mechanical Phlebitis

It is greatly influenced by catheter stiffness and size.

Larger SR catheters are required for same lumen size, and larger Fr catheter sizes cause more mechanical phlebitis than smaller Fr sizes.

SR, however, is less stiff and, therefore, less traumatic to vascular endothelium.

2.6.3   Flow Rates

The flow rate through a capillary is regulated by Poiseuille's law that states that the velocity of a liquid flowing through a capillary is directly proportional to the pressure of the liquid and the fourth power of the radius of the capillary and is inversely proportional to the viscosity of the liquid and the length of the capillary.

So therefore, flows are a function of catheter diameter (to the 4th power) and length.

In the case of catheters with the same Fr size (outer diameter), higher flows are achieved through PUR catheters because they have thinner walls.

2.6.4   Infusate Compatibility

It is a function of catheter composition and structure.

In general, SR is more compatible with infusates, because it is cross-linked and hydrophobic.

It resists hydration and therefore degradation [3].

Alcohols, in particular, can permeate PUR catheters (especially those with polyether soft segments) and carry solubilized drugs with them [9].

2.6.5   Extravasation of Infusates

Extravasation refers to the escape of a drug into the extravascular space, either by leakage from a vessel or by direct infiltration [10].

It can be influenced by catheter and guidewire stiffness, as stiffer catheters/guidewires can puncture the vessel.

Silicone is less stiff, but many guidewires and PUR catheters have soft, flexible "atraumatic" tips to minimize damage to tissue.

This is a major issue for neonates and, in general, minor issue with PICCs.

2.6.6   Catheter Occlusion

Typically catheter obstruction caused by precipitates is a function of the infusates or the administration of incompatible infusates and is not dependent on catheter material properties.

SR catheters of same Fr size as PUR catheters have smaller internal diameter that are more easily blocked by precipitates.

However, PUR is more prone to degradation if alcohol or other solvents are used to dissolve the precipitate [11].

2.6.7   Clotting and Thrombosis

Such complications are influenced by material chemical, as well as physical, properties.

Catheters with greater surface roughness are more thrombogenic (radiopaque barium sulfate filler can have an influence).

Many studies about this topic are not controlled well enough.

Different PURs have varying degrees of resistance to degradation by enzymes and hydrolysis. Polycarbonate-based formulations are more stable than polyether-based polycarbonates.

2.6.8   Catheter Weakening and Embolization

It is related to the stability of the catheter to infusates (including solubilizing agents), disinfectants and cleaning solutions, and biologic environment.

PUR is inherently stronger (higher burst and tensile strength) but is more susceptible to in vivo degradation and attack by solvents.

When the catheter is only used as blood access, PUR is superior.

For drug administration, the use must be decided on a case-by-case basis, heeding manufacturer's warnings.

2.6.9   Vascular Damage

It is a function of catheter stiffness, especially of its tip.

Silicone is softer and less traumatic than PUR, in general; however, thicker catheters are stiffer than thinner catheters.

2.6.10   Catheter Maintenance Requirements

Polyether PURs are subject to degradation by alcohols and disinfectants, especially ointments in a PEG (polyethylene glycol) base.

SR is more resistant to attack by cleaning and disinfecting agents but is more easily torn.

2.7 New Materials

More catheters with coatings containing drugs will be soon available.

The surface of the catheter determines its biological response. Modifications of the surface or release of drugs (e.g., antibiotics, heparin) into the immediate environment can improve biological function without affecting bulk material properties.

The current ideal catheter would have SR's biocompatibility with PUR's mechanical strength. Sil-PUR copolymers have been polymerized and demonstrate promising characteristics.

Polymers with surface-modifying end groups have also been developed, but the difficulty lies in demonstrating clinical utility of new designs and materials. Because the incidence of complications is relatively low, a large sample size is necessary in order to demonstrate a statistical improvement.

2.8 Final Recommendations

1. Deep knowledge of your material and its weaknesses and strengths.
2. Silicones more chemical resistant than polyurethanes.
3. Polyurethanes offer "better" physical properties for access.
4. Not all polyurethanes created equal.
5. Ask for data where applicable.
6. Always look at manufacturer's warnings.

References

1. Ratner BD, Hoffman AS, Schoen FJ, Lemons JE (2013) Biomaterials science. An introduction to materials in medicine. Academic Press (an imprint of Elsevier), Amsterdam
2. Kipping FS (1904) Organic derivative of silicon. Preparation of alkysilicon chlorides. Proc Chem Soc 20:15
3. Di Fiore A. (2007), Polyurethanes in vascular access: clinical perspectives. 21st annual AVA conference, Phoenix, Arizona
4. Degarmo EP, Black JT, Kohser RA (2003) Materials and processes in manufacturing, 9th edn. Wiley, New York
5. Smith WF, Hashemi J (2006) Foundations of materials science and engineering, 4th edn. McGraw-Hill, New York
6. Williams DF (1999) The Williams dictionary of Biomaterials. Liverpool University Press, Liverpool
7. Dorland's Illustrated Medical Dictionary, 32nd Edition, Elsevier Inc.
8. Williams DF (2008) On the mechanisms of biocompatibility. Biomaterials 29(20): 2941–2942

9. Phil Triolo (2005) RAC material properties of polyurethane and silicone catheters: effects on catheter performance vascular access. Workshop Bambino Gesù Hospital, Rome, April 2005
10. Fischer D, Knobf M, Durivage H (1997) The cancer chemotherapy handbook. Mosby, St. Louis, p 514
11. Crnich CJ (2005) The effects of prolonged ethanol exposure on the mechanical properties of polyurethane and silicone catheters used for intravascular access. Infect Control Hosp Epidemiol 26(8):708–714

Vessel Health and Preservation: The Proactive Approach

3

Paul L. Blackburn

3.1 The Traditional Approach

A 52-year-old male is admitted to the emergency department (ED). The patient presents with a low-grade fever (37.2C), generalized muscle aches, pain, swelling, and erythema of the left ankle. Upon closer inspection, there appears to be an open wound over the fibula. When questioned, the patient describes the ankle injury as being a simple abrasion received when he was rock climbing approximately 14 days earlier. The abrasion has been healing but in the past few days has become increasingly painful, warm to touch, and red in color. The ED physician orders a peripheral IV of D5W at 125 ml per hour and the collection of drainage from the site for a wound culture. The ED nurse places an 18-gauge peripheral IV in the patient's right antecubital fossa. The patient is admitted to the hospital for observation.

Forty-eight hours later, the culture results are positive for *Staphylococcus aureus*. The patient is sent for a computed tomography scan which reveals a lytic center with a ring of sclerosis near the distal end of the fibula. A diagnosis of osteomyelitis is confirmed. The attending physician orders vancomycin 500 mg IV every 6 h. The patient has been receiving maintenance fluids through the PIV for the past 48 h. The IV site looks good, showing no signs of redness or swelling; however, the PIV is bothersome to the patient due to its location. The fluids are infusing as prescribed and a good blood return is obtained. The vancomycin is prepared according to manufacturer's guidelines and administered as ordered. During the second dose of vancomycin, the patient complains of pain and tenderness at the IV site. The nurse administering the drug notes redness and tenderness at the IV site. The IV is discontinued and restarted in the left lower arm cephalic vein. The vancomycin infusion continues. Within 24 h, this site also becomes reddened and painful. The IV is removed and restarted in the left antecubital fossa. After a few doses, the IV must

P.L. Blackburn, BSN, MNA, RN, VA-BC
Vice President of Clinical Affairs, Interrad Medical, Inc.,
181 Cheshire Lane, Suite 100, Plymouth, MN 55441, USA
e-mail: pblackburn@interradmedical.com

S. Sandrucci, B. Mussa (eds.), *Peripherally Inserted Central Venous Catheters*,
DOI 10.1007/978-88-470-5665-7_3, © Springer-Verlag Italia 2014

be restarted once again. After 5 days of therapy, the nurse is no longer able to find a vessel that will accept a peripheral IV. The patient is then referred to the hospital's vascular access team (VAT) by his physician. The VAT reviews the patient's chart for relevant information and then assesses the patient's vasculature. A decision is made to place a peripherally inserted central catheter (PICC) in the patient's right upper arm basilic vein. Although challenging, the PICC is placed, tip position confirmed, and therapy continued. The patient is later discharged home for his remaining therapy.

Summary: A reactive approach to IV therapy resulted in multiple peripheral IV sticks for this patient, venous exhaustion in both lower arms, delay in therapy, and a prolonged stay in the hospital. A proactive approach would have resulted in a single peripheral IV, being replaced with a PICC as soon as the diagnosis had been confirmed and a course of therapy decided upon.

3.2 The Proactive Approach

The proactive approach to vessel health and preservation requires a multidisciplinary team evaluation of the patient, the patient's vasculature, and the planned therapy. While somewhat challenging to implement, this approach results in vessel preservation, on time therapy, and improved patient outcomes.

The first step in the process is determining the prescribed therapy and its duration. One of the most important factors to be considered in this phase is the pH and osmolality of the drug to be infused.

3.2.1 Drug pH

Intravenous drugs are represented as an acid or base on the pH scale. Solution characteristics are represented by the pH, which is the hydrogen ion concentration present in a solution. A pH of 7.0 is considered to be neutral. A low pH (below 7.0) represents an acidic concentration, and a high pH (above 7.0) represents a base concentration. The drug is considered more acidic as it approaches zero on the pH scale, and the closer to 14.0, the more alkaline the drug. Blood is slightly alkaline with a pH of approximately 7.4. Extremely alkaline/acidic infusates such as those with a pH less than 5.0 or greater than 9.0 damage the endothelial lining of the vein wall and cause vein irritation. This cascade of damage is the precursor for phlebitis, infiltration, and/or extravasation (refer Table 3.1) [1, 2].

3.2.2 Drug Osmolality

Osmol is a standard unit of osmotic pressure. It is the weight in grams of a solute, existing in a solution as molecules. Osmolality is defined as the number of milliosmols per kilogram of solute. A solution is considered to be hypotonic if the

Table 3.1 Drug pH scale [3, 4]

pH	Scale	Examples
Below 7.0	Acid	Vancomycin (2.4–4.5)
		Doxycycline (1.8–3.3)
		Dopamine (2.5–5.0)
7.0	Neutral	Ceftriaxone (6.6–6.7)
Above 7.0	Alkaline (base)	Acyclovir (10.5–11.6)
		Phenytoin (12.0)

osmolality is below 250 mOsm/L [5]. Examples of hypotonic solutions include sterile water with an osmolality of zero mOsm/L and 0.45 sodium chloride (half-strength saline) with an osmolality of 155 mOsm/L. Hypotonic solutions lower the osmotic pressure, causing fluid to invade the cells. In severe cases, the cells may become swollen and burst. Water intoxication and death may occur [6]. For this reason, hypotonic solutions are not usually suitable infusates alone for volume replacement; however, hypotonic diluents may be used to dilute extremely hypertonic admixtures, making them more hemocompatible and reducing the risks for chemically induced phlebitis or thrombophlebitis [7]. As an example, 0.45 % sodium chloride has an osmolality of approximately 155 mOsm/L.

Blood in the human body is isotonic with an osmolality of 285 mOsm/L. In general, isotonic solutions range from 250 to 350 mOsm/L. Isotonic solutions are less irritating to the endothelial lining of the vein wall. Example: cefazolin sodium one gram in 50 ml of 0.9 % sodium chloride has a final admixture osmolality of 344 mOsm/L [8].

A hypertonic solution has an osmolality of 375 mOsm/L and above [9]. Peripheral parenteral nutrition (PPN) is a good example of a hypertonic solution. The osmolality of PPN is about 750 mOsm/L and above. Infusion of extremely hypertonic solutions into small peripheral veins often results in a chemically induced phlebitis. When a hypertonic solution such as PPN is infused, the tunica intima (inner layer of the vein wall) tries to protect the vein from damage. The body attempts to adjust the drug and blood back to isotonicity. This causes the water to move from the cells of the endothelial layer of the vein wall (tunica intima) to the infusate in the blood, resulting in shrinkage and dehydration of the cells of the endothelial layer. Subsequent doses may result in further insult to the intima resulting in phlebitis, thrombophlebitis, infiltration, extravasation, sclerosis, and pain [10].

According to the 2011 Infusion Nursing Standards of Practice, infusates with a final admixture osmolality exceeding 600 mOsm/L require administration via a central venous catheter [11].

Examples [12, 13]:

Infusate	Osmolality
Cefazolin sodium 1 g in 20 mL 0.9 % sodium chloride	426 mOsm/L
4o mEq potassium + D5W and 0.9 % sodium chloride solution	642 mOsm/L
10 % calcium chloride	2,102 mOsm/L
Dextrose 50 % in water (D50W)	2,526 mOsm/L

Note: Nutritional solutions with final concentrations exceeding 10 % dextrose and/or 5 % amino acids should be administered through a central venous catheter with the tip terminating in the lower one-third of the superior vena cava (SVC) to the junction of the SVC and the right atrium. For lower extremity insertion sites, the catheter tip should reside in the thoracic inferior vena cava (IVC) above the level of the diaphragm [14].

Some drugs may cause insult to the venous endothelium as a result of their inherent chemical structure. Although these drugs may be isotonic and have a relatively neutral pH, they may still irritate the venous endothelium and induce phlebitis and thrombophlebitis. Drug examples in this category include nafcillin and erythromycin. Nafcillin and erythromycin are inherently irritating drugs and are often associated with a higher incidence of chemical phlebitis and infiltration [15].

Summary: Hemodilution of the drug pH is crucial to reducing complications associated with infusion of extremely acidic or alkaline drugs. Clinical research has shown that drugs with a pH below 4.1 and above 9.0 cause endothelial damage to the intima of the vein [16]. According to the 2011 Infusion Nursing Standards of Practice, a central venous catheter is recommended when infusing agents with a pH greater than 9.0 or less than 5.0 [17]. The same is true for drugs with extreme osmolality. Therapies are not appropriate for peripheral infusion with an osmolality greater than 600 mOsm/l [18].

3.2.3 Length of Therapy

The second factor to consider when attempting to be proactive regarding vessel health and preservation is the *length and frequency of the infusion*. The CDC makes the following recommendation in their 2011 Guidelines for the Prevention of Catheter-Related Bloodstream Infections: use a midline catheter or peripherally inserted central catheter (PICC), instead of a short peripheral catheter, when the duration of IV therapy will likely exceed 6 days [19]. The CDC guidelines provide one factor to be considered when selecting a vascular access device. In addition to this factor, medical device manufacturers provide recommendations to guide the safe use of their devices. These guidelines are particular to the device type and construction, as well as recommended dwell time and catheter tip location (see Table 3.2).

The frequency of the infusion must be considered when placing a vascular access device using a proactive approach. The frequency of the infusion may vary based on patient response, type of infusate, or number of doses required. As an example, many antibiotics are infused from one to four times daily, whereas a chemotherapeutic drug may be administered one time every 14 days.

Summary: The length and frequency of therapy play a role in vessel health and preservation. As noted, if the therapy is expected to last longer than 6 days, a device other than a peripheral IV catheter should be placed. The choice of vascular access device is based on both factors. In other words, a PICC may be selected for long-term antibiotic therapy where a port or tunneled CVC may be more appropriate for intermittent chemotherapy administration.

Table 3.2 Recommended VAD insertion sites

Device type	Manufacturer's insertion site recommendation	Standard of practice
PIV	No recommendation	Considered should be given to those veins found on the dorsal and ventral surfaces of the upper extremities, including the metacarpal, cephalic, basilic, and median veins [25]
Midline catheter	Above the antecubital fossa, avoiding areas where catheter may kink[a]	Site selection should be routinely initiated in the region of the antecubital fossa. Veins that should be considered for midline catheter cannulation are the basilic, cephalic, and brachial veins [26]
PICC	Placement above the antecubital fossa is recommended. Avoid placing in areas that could lead to kinking[b]	Veins that should be considered for PICC cannulation are the basilic, median cubital, cephalic, and brachial veins [26]
CVC	Select a vein by assessing patient anatomy and condition. If the subclavian vein is used, the vein is entered percutaneously at the point that identifies the junction of the outer and middle thirds of the clavicle[c]	The subclavian vein is recommended in adult patients, rather than the jugular or femoral veins, although benefits and risks accompany each access site. For patients with chronic kidney disease, the subclavian vein is not recommended in order to preserve the vein [27]
Port	Ports can be placed in the arm or in the chest. Recommended veins for arm placement include cephalic, basilic, or median cubital. Recommended veins for chest placement include internal jugular or lateral subclavian[d]	The clinician should collaborate with the health-care team and patient in the assessment and site selection for placement of implanted ports [27]

[a]Bard Access Systems Polyurethane Midline Catheter Instructions for use
[b]Bard Access Systems PowerPICC SOLO Instructions for use
[c]Bard Access Systems PowerHohn Instructions for use
[d]Bard Access Systems PowerPort Implantable Port Instructions for use

3.2.4 Body Habitus and Comorbidities

Next, the *patient condition* must be taken into account when practicing the proactive approach to vessel health and preservation and vascular access device selection and placement. The clinician should ask the following questions:

1. What was the patient admitted to the hospital for in the first place? A suspected infection might lead the clinician to choose a particular vascular access device, whereas a surgical procedure may lead to an entirely different choice of vascular access device.
2. Does the patient have any comorbidities that may affect the integrity of their vasculature? Comorbidities such as long-term diabetes or steroid use will affect vessel integrity and therefore play a major role in the device selection process. How about obesity? Morbid obesity may affect the size, location, and accessibil-

ity of the vessels a clinician may have to use to provide IV therapy. Is there any evidence of chronic kidney disease? What is the glomerular filtration rate (GFR)? Is this a new condition or a long-term condition? Many hospitals have policies requiring a nephrology consult if the patient is in or nearing chronic renal failure based on the GFR.

3. Does the patient have a history of previous vascular access devices? If so, where (anatomically) was the device placed? How long was the device in place? What type of device was used previously? How many times has this patient had vascular access devices placed previously? Does the patient have a vascular access device in place currently? If so, what type, how long has it been in place, and what is the current patency status of the device?

4. What is the condition of the patient's vasculature? If the patient has had multiple previous vascular access devices, do they have patent vessels in their extremities? Obesity is also a factor to be considered at this time as well as vessels that may be deeper within the anatomy of these individuals and therefore inaccessible for select vascular access devices.

5. Finally, what will the vascular access device be used for? Is it merely for infusion therapy or will the device be used for blood specimen collection? If so, how often?

Assessing patient condition must also take patient activity and device dwell time into account. The patient who is going to be on bed rest for the duration of the therapy may be considered for a particular type of vascular access device, whereas a patient who is ambulatory or will be going home with the device may be considered for another type of vascular access device. Understanding patient activity during the time a vascular access device will dwell may also be affected by the patient's perception of the device and how that device will affect their self-image. A patient who is able to go about their normal daily activities may not want anyone to know they have a vascular access device in place. The placing clinician must understand the effect the vascular access device will have on the patient's cosmesis and take this information into account as well.

Finally, once a preliminary vascular access device decision has been made, the placing clinician should complete a thorough examination of the patient's vasculature. This step often results in a visual inspection as well as an ultrasound inspection of the vessel health and integrity. Vessels that have been previously used for vascular access devices may carry the scars of these previous devices in the form of a partial occlusion. If that is the case or in the event there are other traumas, old injuries, etc., at the proposed insertion site, another site should be selected.

Summary: All aspects of the patient's health status must be taken into account prior to making a preliminary decision upon the vascular device to be placed.

3.2.5   Risk

The *fourth factor* to consider when using the proactive approach to a vascular access device is the considerations around providing a device that represents the lowest risk to the patient. This decision point involves understanding the manufacturer recommendations and the standards of practice surrounding the following:

1. Insertion location of the vascular access device (VAD)
2. Catheter-to-vein ratio
3. VAD material
4. VAD indications

Each vascular access device is provided with the manufacturer's recommendations as to the potential insertion sites for the device and, in some cases, the terminal tip location of the device. Table 3.2 illustrates both the manufacturer's recommendations as well as insertion locations based on the 2011 INS Recommended Standards of Practice. Other societal standards should be reviewed and considered when determining site location as well. Additionally, the site itself should be thoroughly evaluated and the risks associated with that site determined. The site should be free of infection, scarring, or injury. There are also risks associated with particular sites that must be considered. It is well known that femoral insertion sites are generally associated with higher infection rates. Thus, regulatory agencies recommend the use of other insertion sites unless the femoral site is the only alternative. The CDC recommends avoiding the use of the femoral vein for central venous access in adult patients as a category 1A recommendation—the strongest recommendation backed by clinical evidence [20].

Summary: Use manufacturer's recommendations along with evidence-based recommendations from an appropriate society such as the Infusion Nurses Society to make a decision regarding placement of a vascular access device. Additionally, following selection of a device and insertion site, the vessel health as well as the general health of the insertion site must be taken into account.

3.2.6 Infection Risk

When assessing the risk associated with a VAD, the clinician must also take into account the infection rates of particular VADs and the amount of space the catheter will occupy in the patient's vein. The catheter-to-vein ratio may be directly related to upper extremity deep vein thrombosis.

There are over five million CVCs placed in the United States annually [21]. These devices are associated with their share of complications. The first complication that comes to mind is central line-associated infections (CLABSI). It is estimated that 87 % of the CLABSIs occurring in the United States are related to VADs [22]. CLABSI rates can be affected by both the methods used to place the VAD and methods used for care and maintenance of the VAD. Additionally, there seems to be a correlation between the length of dwell time and CLABSI rates. Data also exists validating the insertion risk specifically related to the methods used during insertion, i.e., maximal barrier precautions vs. clean procedure; urgency of the insertion, i.e., VAD inserted at the site of a traumatic accident, or in the emergency department, or in a controlled environment; and the actual insertion site as noted above.

Catheter-related deep vein thrombosis is common with VADs, especially those placed in the upper extremities. A recent study indicated that up to 40 % of these devices lead to asymptomatic thrombosis [23]. Drs. Thomas Nifong and Timothy J. McDevitt recently completed a study using fluid dynamics to calculate relative flow rates as a function of the ratio of the catheter to vein diameter. Dr. Nifong found that "fluid flow is dramatically decreased by the insertion of a centrally located obstruction" [24]. Although this is a laboratory study, it does serve to help the inserting clinician understand the potential issues associated with inserting VADs in human anatomy. There is a very real possibility that the incidence of upper extremity DVT is related to the blood flow, or lack thereof, around a VAD placed in an upper extremity vessel. While no formal recommendations exist, it is evident that the risk of upper extremity DVT is much greater with a PICC than a peripheral IV.

Summary: Catheter-related risks such as infection and thrombosis must be considered when selecting a VAD. These risks must be weighed against the benefits of a particular device to the patient.

3.2.7 VAD Material

Finally, vascular access device materials may also be implicated as a risk to the patient. A thorough understanding of the catheter material and the properties of that material will enable the clinician to make an informed decision about the VAD selection. Today, polyurethane in its many forms and silicone are considered the gold standard when selecting catheter materials. Both fall into a class of material known as polymers. The word polymer derives from the Greek "poly" meaning many and "mer" meaning part. Thus, the word literally means many parts. Polymers are materials made up of smaller molecules that are chemically linked into long chains. These long chains vary in the number and type of molecules used to formulate a specific polymer. Polyurethane VADs are available in many different varieties. These devices, while biocompatible, can be stiff or soft depending upon the molecules that make up the polyurethane chain. Those that contain more "plastic" molecules are generally going to be stiffer and therefore more likely to damage the intimal layer of cells in the vein leading to an increased rate of thrombosis, while those that are softer will be more vein friendly, resulting in lower rates of intimal layer damage. Silicone elastomers are made from long linear dimethylsiloxane-type molecules, which are then reinforced with silica filler and cross-linked. Silicone catheters are soft and flexible and therefore generally cause less damage to the intimal layer of the vein. However, because silicone is softer, silicone catheters are generally thicker to provide additional strength for VADs. Once again, the catheter-to-vein ratio must be considered.

Summary: Catheter material must be considered when assessing the risk of the VAD to the patient. Polyurethane catheters are stronger and will generally last longer; however, due to their structure, they may be harder on the vein lining which can lead to increased rates of thrombosis. Silicone catheters may be more vein friendly but are generally larger in diameter to account for the soft material. In both cases, the diameter of the catheter must be considered in relationship to the diameter of the proposed insertion vein in its resting state.

Conclusion

A proactive approach to vessel health and preservation is essential in the healthcare arena of the twenty-first century. This chapter discusses the many factors that must be taken into account when considering a vascular access device for the individual patient. The discussion would not be complete without understanding the basic model that must be used when making a patient care decision. The model is based on three variables:

1. The patient
2. The clinician and their practice
3. The medical device or product

These variables interact with each other to ultimately affect the patient outcome. Each must be given equal weight when considering the need for a VAD and the type of VAD chosen. This chapter has presented many of the variables associated with the patient, the practice, and the product. Take the proactive approach to vessel health by clearly evaluating all of the variables involved and their impact on the expected outcome.

References

1. Hankins J (2010) Anatomy and physiology related to infusion therapy. In: Alexander M, Corrigan A, Gorski L, Hankins J, Perucca R (eds) Infusion nursing: an evidence-based approach (3rd ed, pp. 178–203), 3rd edn. Saunders, St. Louis, p 187
2. Perucca R (2010) Peripheral venous access devices. In: Alexander M, Corrigan A, Gorski L, Hankins J, Perucca R (eds) Infusion nursing: an evidence-based approach (3rd ed, pp. 456–479). Saunders, St. Louis, p 474
3. Kokotis K (1998) Preventing chemical phlebitis. Nursing 28(11):42–46, pp. 43
4. Kokotis K (1998) Preventing chemical phlebitis. Nursing 28(11):42–46, pp. 44
5. Phillips L (2010) Parenteral fluids. In: Alexander M, Corrigan A, Gorski L, Hankins J, Perucca R (eds) Infusion nursing: an evidence-based approach (3rd ed, pp. 229–241). Saunders, St. Louis, p 233
6. Weinstein SM (2007) Plumer's principles and practice of intravenous therapy, 8th edn. Lippincott, Philadelphia, p 130, 136
7. Kokotis K (1998) Preventing chemical phlebitis. Nursing 28(11):42–46, p. 42
8. Kokotis K (1998) Preventing chemical phlebitis. Nursing 28(11):42–46, pp. 42, 44
9. Phillips L (2010) Parenteral fluids. In: Alexander M, Corrigan A, Gorski L, Hankins J, Perucca R (eds) Infusion nursing: an evidence-based approach (3rd ed, pp. 229–241). Saunders, St. Louis, p 233
10. Kokotis K (1998) Preventing chemical phlebitis. Nursing 28(11):42–46, p. 44
11. Infusion Nurses Society (2011) Infusion nurses standards of practice. J Infus Nurs 34(1S): S37, S38, S92
12. Kokotis K (1998) Preventing chemical phlebitis. Nursing 28(11):42–46, p. 42
13. Kokotis K (1998) Preventing chemical phlebitis. Nursing 28(11):42–46, p. 43
14. Infusion Nurses Society (2011) Infusion nurses standards of practice. J Infus Nurs 34(1S):S45
15. Kokotis K (1998) Preventing chemical phlebitis. Nursing 28(11):42–46, pp. 44–45

16. Kokotis K (1998) Preventing chemical phlebitis. Nursing 28(11):42–46, pp. 42
17. Infusion Nurses Society (2011) Infusion nurses standards of practice. J Infus Nurs 34(1S):S37, S38
18. Infusion Nurses Society (2011) Infusion nurses standards of practice. J Infus Nurs 34(1S):37
19. O'Grady N (2011) Guidelines for the prevention of intravascular catheter-related infections. Centers for Disease Control and Prevention. MMWR Recomm Rep.
20. CDC Recommendations for the reduction of catheter-related blood stream infections (2011). p. 11
21. McGee DC, Gould MK (2003) Preventing complications of central venous catheterization. N Engl J Med 348:1123–1133
22. Dariouiche R (2001) Device associated infections: A macroproblem that starts with a micro-adherence. Clinical Infectious Diseases 33:1567–1572
23. Abullah BJ et al (2005) Incidence of upper limb venous thrombosis associated with peripher-ally inserted central catheters (PICC). Br J Radiol 798(931):596–600
24. Nifong T et al (2011) The effect of catheter to vein ratio on blood flow rates in a simulated model of peripherally inserted central venous catheters. Chest 104(1):48–53
25. Infusion Nurses Society (2011) Infusion nurses standards of practice. J Infus Nurs 34: S40–S41
26. Infusion Nurses Society (2011) Infusion nurses standards of practice. J Infus Nurs 34:S41
27. Infusion Nurses Society (2011) Infusion nurses standards of practice. J Infus Nurs 34:S42

The Choice of a Vein in Critically Ill Patients: Cost-Effectiveness

4

Massimo Lamperti

4.1 The Critically Ill Patient

The classical definition of critically ill patients or acutely critical patients refers to patients with one or more impaired vital organ functions such that there is a high probability of imminent or life-threatening deterioration in the patient's condition. Such a definition can also be extended to any patient with any severe chronic disease (e.g., end-stage diabetes, severe heart/renal/liver failure) impairing vital signs. At this stage, a highly complex decision process is necessary to stabilize and support vital organ functions and avoid further deterioration of the clinical conditions.

Even oncological patients can be considered critically ill as their vital organs can be critically damaged by prolonged chemotherapy or progression of their neoplasm.

All these patients usually need a venous access in order to restore hypovolemia, for administration of drugs and parenteral nutrition, and to allow multiple blood samplings.

The choice of the vein to cannulate is crucial in critically ill patients because the veins' patrimony is reduced; the patient could be hypovolemic and with peripheral vascular constriction and sometimes the intravenous access has to be achieved in emergency for rapid volume infusion.

Peripheral veins are usually cannulated for the administration of drugs and fluids. Although they are used during the early resuscitation phase for rapid infusion of high volumes of fluids, they could fail due to extravasation. Central venous cannulation is the preferred route of administration of large volumes of fluids, low/high pH drugs, high osmolarity drugs, or drugs causing intimal damage, and it can be used to allow hemodynamic monitoring or when peripheral veins are no longer available.

M. Lamperti
Department of Anesthesiology, Cleveland Clinic Abu Dhabi,
Al Maryah Island, Abu Dhabi, UAE
e-mail: docmassimomd@gmail.com

S. Sandrucci, B. Mussa (eds.), *Peripherally Inserted Central Venous Catheters*, 31
DOI 10.1007/978-88-470-5665-7_4, © Springer-Verlag Italia 2014

The subclavian vein has for years been considered the central vein of choice in critically ill patients because its cannulation is related to a reduced rate of thrombosis and catheter-related infections [1]. However, this procedure is highly affected by major mechanical complications (e.g., pneumothorax, arterial puncture, hemothorax), and to avoid them, a skilled operator is mandatory [2].

Other central veins commonly used in critically patients are the internal jugular vein and the femoral vein, given their relative increased size and the possibility to avoid life-threatening complications in case of inadvertent puncture of the nearby arteries (in case of femoral vein cannulation). For these reasons, the femoral vein has been suggested as the preferred site of central venous cannulation in case of emergencies with an unknown coagulation state [3], and to promptly remove this access when full restoration of vital signs has been reached, coagulation state is checked and a secure central vein catheter is placed in the internal jugular or subclavian vein.

The use of peripheral deep veins to place central venous catheters started in the early 1970s with the introduction of Drum Cartridge catheters [4]. These catheters had a low success after their initial introduction in the clinical setting due to a higher rate of mechanical complications such as hematomas and thrombosis. Complications were related to the large-bore needle used for vein puncture causing major endothelial damage, the use of a blind technique, and the lack of the vessels' measurement before catheter placement.

The introduction of ultrasound guidance, new polyurethane, and power-injectable peripheral-inserted central venous catheters (PICCs) [5–8] allowed the reduction of the main complications and the possibility of the administration of high volumes of fluids even in the critical acute patient.

4.2   Physiology of the Venous Flow

Hemodynamics of the vessel is governed by a variety of physical properties and laws that explain blood flow through the vascular system. The main mechanism promoting venous return during normal motory activity is the muscle pump system. Peripheral veins have one-way valves that direct flow away from the limb and toward the heart. Veins physically located within large muscle groups undergo compression as the muscles surrounding them contract, and they become decompressed as the muscles relax. Therefore, with normal cycles of contraction and relaxation, the veins are alternately compressed and decompressed. Muscle contraction propels blood forward through the open distal valves and impedes flow into the muscle as the proximal valves close during contraction. During muscle relaxation, the proximal valves open and blood flows into and fills the venous segment. Initially during relaxation, the distal valves close, but then they open as the volume of blood and pressure increases in the venous segment. The net effect is that the cycle of compression and relaxation propels the blood in the direction of the heart. Venous valves prevent the blood from flowing backwards, thereby permitting unidirectional flow that enhances venous return.

Normal venous return can be impaired in the case of venous flow reduction as it can happen in the case of venous cannulation. Under normal conditions, two major mechanisms in the body operate to prevent venous hypertension. First, bicuspid valves in the veins prevent backflow and venous pooling. Deep venous thrombosis (DVT) commonly occurs at these valves, causing irreversible damage to the valve. Second, during normal motion, muscles decrease venous pressures by approximately 40 % in the upper extremities. With rest, pressures return to normal in approximately 30 s. In diseased veins or when a vein is cannulated with a large-bore catheter whose diameter occupies more than 50 % of the inner cross-sectional diameter of the vein, movement decreases venous pressures by only 20 %. In this latter case, the hemodynamic changes in the venous flow enhance a hypercoagulability state that contributes to thrombosis. Recent studies have shown that the incidence of symptomatic catheter-related thrombosis (CRT) is <5 %, whereas the incidence of asymptomatic CRT is higher, at 14–18 % [9–11].

The two major consequences of DVT are pulmonary embolism (PE) and post-phlebitic syndrome.

PE supervenes when a clot dislodges and travels through the inferior vena cava and right heart chambers, finally reaching and obstructing a portion of the pulmonary vasculature. PE is common (incidence of approximately 600,000 per year in the United States) and is often fatal, with an untreated mortality rate of 30–40 %.

In order to define if a vein is still able to maintain its normal flow, two main diagnostic techniques can be performed: compression ultrasound (CUS) and venous compression duplex ultrasonography.

CUS is a variation of the commonly used medical ultrasound technique, in which sound waves are applied to the tissue by means of a probe, and an image of the tissue is constructed from the returning sound waves [12–14]. With compression ultrasound, the ultrasound probe is placed over the suspected vein, and an ultrasound image of the vein is produced, as is typically done with ultrasound techniques. The operator then attempts to compress the vein by pushing on it with the ultrasound probe.

Veins are typically highly compressible; in other words, veins can be collapsed temporarily by applying pressure to them. But if DVT is present, it is relatively difficult to collapse the vein because of the presence of a blood clot, so its compressibility is reduced. When a vein is noncompressible, that is a reliable indicator that DVT is present [12].

Compression ultrasonography has both high sensitivity and specificity for detecting proximal deep vein thrombosis only in symptomatic patients [13, 14].

Venous compression duplex ultrasonography is a readily available noninvasive technique that is 95 % sensitive for the diagnosis of symptomatic DVT in a proximal vein but only 75 % sensitive for diagnosing symptomatic deep peripheral veins thrombi. This technique uses real-time ultrasound scanning to image the vein and pulsed Doppler ultrasound to assess blood flow within it [8].

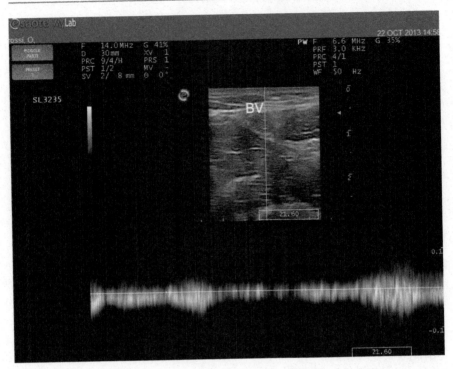

Fig. 4.1 Normal venous flow in the basilic vein (*BV*). The venous flow seems pulsatile because the cardiac pulsatility of the brachial artery transduces its pulsation to the nearby structures

Criteria used for diagnosis of DVT with duplex ultrasonography include the inability to compress the vein with direct pressure (suggesting the presence of an intraluminal thrombus), direct visualization of the thrombus, and absence of blood flow within the vessel (Figs. 4.1 and 4.2).

4.3 Assessment of Cost-Effectiveness During Venous Cannulation Choice

Cost-effectiveness analysis (CEA) is a form of economic analysis that compares the relative costs and outcomes (effects) of two or more courses of action. Cost-effectiveness analysis is distinct from cost-benefit analysis, which assigns a monetary value to the measure of effect [15].

Typically, the CEA is expressed in terms of a ratio where the denominator is a gain in health from a measure (e.g., years of life) and the numerator is the cost associated with the health gain [16]. The most commonly used outcome measure is quality-adjusted life years (QALY) [17]. Cost-effectiveness analyses are often visualized on a cost-effectiveness plane consisting of four quadrants. Outcomes plotted in Quadrant I are more effective and more expensive, those in Quadrant II are more

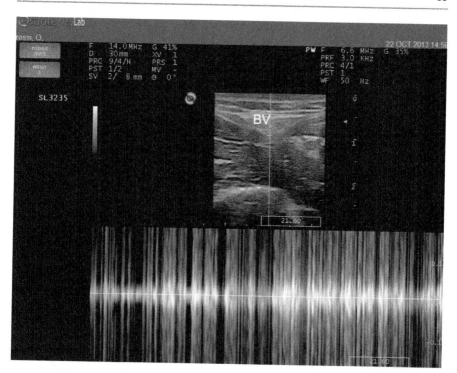

Fig. 4.2 Reduced venous flow in the brachial vein (*BV*). The slow amplitude pulsatile waveforms reveal a reduced flow. This could be normal when the vein is compressed during skin compression or when the vein has a reduced flow as in thrombosis

effective and less expensive, those in Quadrant III are less effective and less expensive, and those in Quadrant IV are less effective and more expensive [18].

In order to apply the CEA during the choice of the vein and of the catheter, some objective factors (possibility of administration of any drug, availability of the vein, risk of mechanical complications, risk of infectious complications) such as subjective factors (acceptance by the patient, comfort of the patient, pain due to vein cannulation) should be considered. In particular, the QALY related to the use of a specific device (in this case, the central venous catheter) is expressed as the improvement in the patient's quality of life measured as:

- Time trade-off: patient is asked if he/she preferred to have the device and spending the rest of his/her life with this device or not having the device but having a shorter lifespan.
- Standard gamble: patient is asked if he/she preferred not to insert the device or insert the device with the gambling of having/not having a better health condition.
- Rating scale: patients are asked to rate the device according a 0–10 score.

The choice of the vein starts from the choice of the catheter. A simplified algorithm (Fig. 4.3) can guide the choice of the catheter according to the patient's clinical conditions.

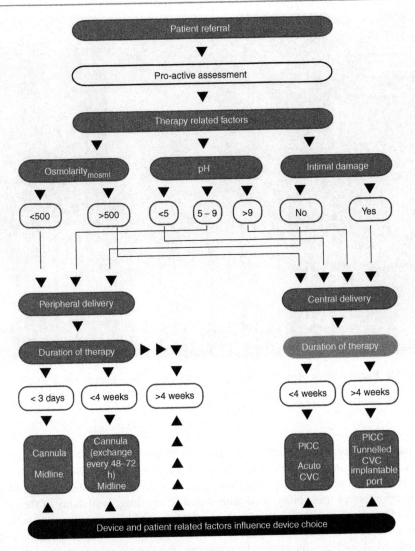

Fig. 4.3 Algorithm for choosing the vein

The choice of the vein for PICC insertion has to follow rules similar to the other vascular devices according to the anatomical measurements and findings discovered after a preliminary ultrasound examination of the arm and patient's physical conditions.

The major contraindications for PICC insertion related to patients' conditions are:

1. Reduced movement of the arm, where the PICC has to be inserted (paresis or reduced motility caused by temporary inability (fracture of the arm))
2. Ipsilateral axillary lymphoadenectomy
3. Skin infection over the insertion site
4. Skin burns or skin altered over the insertion site
5. Patients with possible future needs for an arteriovenous fistula

A minor contraindication for inserting a PICC line in the arm is represented by the possibility to visualize the vein to cannulate in one of its two main planes

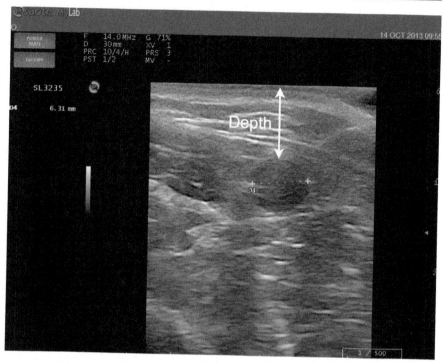

Fig. 4.4 Vein depth in short axis view. The *arrow marks* the distance between the skin and the anterior wall of the basilic vein

(longitudinal or transversal). In this latter case, if this vein represents the only possible solution, the operator inserting the catheter should pay more attention in order to avoid inadvertent puncture of important structures surrounding the vein.

4.3.1   How to Choose the Correct Vein

This analysis is focused mainly on PICC line insertion even if these general concepts could be extended to any vessel to be cannulated.

Brachial veins and basilic veins are the main veins used for PICC line insertion. The cephalic vein is not used routinely as it is usually too superficial, and when it enters the axillary vein, a very acute angle is created so that the passage of the guide wire and even that of the catheter could be difficult. Cephalic veins are usually deeper in obese patients, but their cannulation should be considered as a second choice given their tendency to collapse that could favor vein thrombosis.

4.3.1.1 Vein Depth

Vein depth has to be measured during the ultrasound examination of the deep vessels in the arm. This distance has to be calculated freezing the ultrasound image in a transversal and longitudinal plane and measuring it from the skin surface to the anterior wall of the vein (Figs. 4.4 and 4.5). This measurement allows the operator to avoid a deeper entrance of the needle into the skin in case the vein is

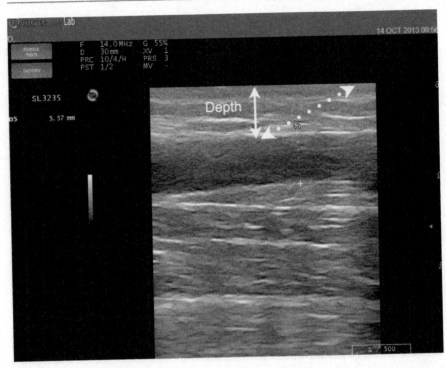

Fig. 4.5 Vein depth in longitudinal axis view. The *arrow marks* the distance between the skin and the anterior wall of the vein while the *dotted arrow marks* the distance the needle has to do from skin puncture to vein puncture. This distance could help the operator in order to avoid inadvertent posterior vein wall puncture in an in-plane approach

very superficial or to use a longer needle in case the vein is very deep as in severe obese patients.

4.3.1.2 Cross-Sectional Diameter
Another important standard for a correct choice of the vein is the cross-sectional diameter. This can be measured both in the transversal and the longitudinal axis. In the transversal view, the cross-sectional diameter is measured from the left lateral to the right lateral wall (Fig. 4.6), while in the longitudinal view, the cross-sectional diameter is measured from the anterior to the posterior wall of the vein (Fig. 4.7). This latter diameter is usually reduced than transversal cross-sectional diameter. The best predictor for catheter and vein choice is the cross-sectional area, an automatically calculated measure that is calculated taking into consideration several cross-sectional diameters. The cross-sectional area of a vessel multiplied by the velocity (cm/s) at that point gives the blood flow value (ml/s) at that level. For this reason, the flow of the vein is better represented by the cross-sectional diameter. An important issue is not to impair venous flow inserting a large-bore catheter whose diameter can be too big or even the same of the cross-sectional diameter itself.

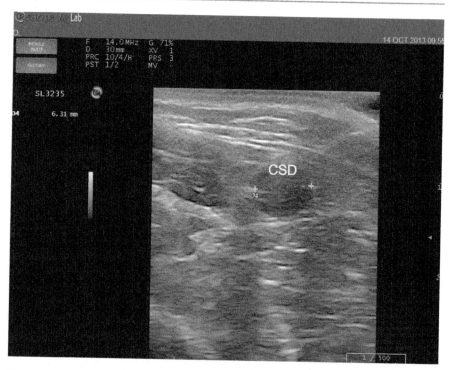

Fig. 4.6 Cross-sectional diameter (*CSD*) of the vein in a short axis view. The measurement reveals a 6.31 mm diameter in the basilic vein

4.3.1.3 Catheter Vein Ratio

The Infusion Nurses Society recommended in 2006 that a target vein for access must be able to accommodate the catheter, but no specific size guidelines were stated [18]. An in vitro study [19] demonstrated the specific impact of catheters on fluid flow rates and suggested a common rule to apply when choice of catheter has to be performed. Even this was only a mathematical model, and a true venous system has a more complex pulsatile flow; through parallel, branching vein systems with curving and tapering veins capable of adaptive variations, it could predict in vivo conditions. Branch points may create local areas of turbulence, but overall laminar flow conditions would be maintained even in a complex venous system. Despite that, veins include curves and angulations. Fluid dynamics predict that curves reduce flow rates as compared with straight cylinders, and the effect of catheterization would depend on the catheter location. If the catheter followed the outer radius of the curve, the highest velocity portion of the cylinder would be obstructed and the effect would be similar to that of a straight segment with a centrally placed catheter. Veins are normally tapered, with a gradually increasing diameter. An increasing cylinder diameter would decrease the obstructive effect on the relative flow rate. For example, with an initial catheter-to-vein ratio of 0:3, in case of a

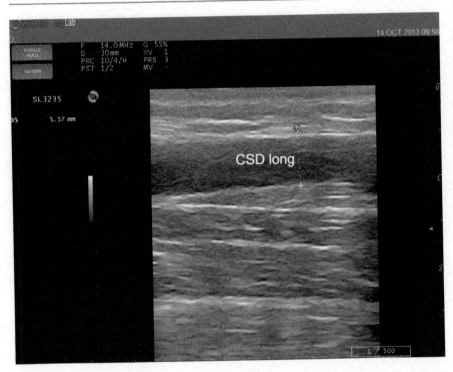

Fig. 4.7 Cross-sectional diameter of the vein in longitudinal axis (CSD long). The measurement reveals a 5.57 diameter in the same basilic vein as in Fig. 4.6. The ellipsoidal shape and the elastic properties of the veins cause this difference between the CSD and the CSD long

vein's diameter increase by 10 % over the length of the system, the relative flow would be 0.38 rather than 0.30.

Veins are distensible, but partial obstruction of a single vein in the upper extremity would result in only a modest pressure change. It is unlikely that a partially obstructed vein would have a major vasodilatation based on this pressure change.

PICCs in particular may substantially decrease venous flow rates likely due in part to the greater impact on blood flow.

Given these "in vitro" results, the suggested catheter-vein ratio threshold in order to avoid venous thrombosis has been established to be 0.3 (Fig. 4.6). In example, a basilic vein whose cross-sectional diameter is 6 mm can be safely cannulated with a 6F (2 mm outer catheter diameter) PICC.

4.3.1.4 Exit Site

The exit site of PICCs should be in the central part of the arm [20]. This site is far away from airway secretions, in an area where the skin is particularly dry and less contaminated. Any puncture of the vein near the elbow or the shoulder should not be used to avoid an excessive flexion of the catheter or an increased risk of infection due to sweating. A problem would arise if the vein to be punctured in this area has reduced sizes that could increase the risk of thrombosis (e.g., reduced catheter/vein ratio) or the vein is near to dangerous structures and its cannulation could increase the risk of major complications as nerve puncture or arterial puncture. In this latter situation, the choice of the vein could be different: the vein could be punctured more cranially (even at the axilla), but the exit site of the catheter could be moved to the central part of the arm by a tunneling procedure. PICCs' tunneling cannot be suggested as a routine procedure and before achieving an appropriate competence. Further studies are needed to demonstrate its real benefit on the reduction of infections and better tolerance for patients.

4.3.2 Clinical Scenarios

Case 1. A 75-year-old obese male patient was admitted to the ICU after oncological colorectal surgery. A short-term central venous line was placed perioperatively (7F-2lumen) in the internal jugular vein. Just after his admission in the ICU, the patient suffered from postoperative delirium and accidentally removed the central line catheter. The nurse received orders from doctors regarding vancomycin infusion, parenteral nutrition, and monitoring of the central venous oxygen saturation (ScVO2). The patient was hemodynamically stable, he was extubated just at the end of the surgery, and he was able to move his arms.

The nurse in charge calls the doctor on-call and asked for a central venous catheter placement order. The doctor was not able to place central lines by using ultrasound guidance. He called the vascular specialist, who first of all asked why the patient needed a central line and started an ultrasound examination of the vessels at the arm and the thorax. The ultrasound examination showed a large basilic vein (cross-sectional diameter 6.8 mm) 2 cm deep. There were also two small brachial veins very near to the artery. The basilic vein had a straight pathway till its confluence with the brachial veins. The axillary vein was compressible and it was visible till its entrance in the subclavian vein. The cephalic vein was superficial (depth 1 cm) and easily compressible.

The vascular specialist in this case chose to cannulate the basilic vein with a 6F double lumen PICC in order to reduce the thrombotic risk and to use ultrasound guidance followed by an intracavitary electrocardiogram in order to properly place the tip of the catheter at the atrium.

The vein was successfully placed and the catheter was used to administer antibiotics and nutrition. A blood sample taken from the catheter revealed a good mixed-venous oxygenation meaning a good metabolic state.

Case 2. A 32-year-old lady was scheduled for long-term antibiotic therapy caused by a bone fracture infection. She received the therapy initially by mouth, but because of antibiotic resistance, her doctor ordered a 6 months therapy for her. She was admitted into an outpatient center where she was visited. The infusion nurse suggested the placement of a long-term catheter to the patient explaining the possibility to place a port catheter or a PICC line. The patient preferred to have the PICC line, as she was needle-phobic. An ultrasound examination of her vessels in the arm was performed. Her basilic vein had reduced diameters in the right arm while the left basilic vein was 4.4 mm in its cross-sectional diameter and the brachial veins had 3.1 mm cross-sectional diameters bilaterally with overlap with the brachial artery. The infusion nurse chose to puncture the left basilic vein and inserting a 4F PICC single-lumen line with a power-injectable catheter. This solution allowed the patient to receive the antibiotic intermittently and to use the catheter during angio-MRI examinations she had to perform during her clinical history. At the end of this 6 months period, the patient fully recovered from her infection and the PICC line was removed without any problem.

References

1. Merrer J, De Jonghe B, Golliot F et al (2001) Complications of femoral and subclavian venous catheterization in critically ill patients: a randomized controlled trial. JAMA 286:700–707
2. McGee DC, Gould MK (2003) Preventing complications of central venous catheterization. N Engl J Med 348:1123–1133
3. American College of Emergency Physicians policy statement: emergency ultrasound guidelines. American College of Emergency Physicians Web site. Available at: http://www.acep.org/WorkArea/DownloadAsset.aspx?id=32878. Accessed 15th Oct 2013
4. Marsh R, Campbell N (2007) Drum cartridge catheter. Anaesthesia 40:604
5. Neuman M, Murphy B, Rosen M (2006) Bedside placement of peripherally inserted central catheters: a cost-effectiveness analysis. Radiology 206:424–428
6. Galloway M (2010) Insertion and placement of central catheters in the oncology patient. Semin Oncol Nurs 26:102–112
7. Tariq M, Huang D (2006) PICCing the best access for your patient. Crit Care 10:315
8. Selis J, Kadakia S (2009) Venous Doppler sonography of the extremities: a window to pathology of the thorax, abdomen, and pelvis. AJR Am J Roentgenol 193:1446–1451
9. Muñoz F, Mismetti P, Poggio R et al (2008) Clinical outcome of patients with upper-extremity deep vein thrombosis: results from the RIETE Registry. Chest 133:143
10. Kucher N (2011) Clinical practice. Deep-vein thrombosis of the upper extremities. N Engl J Med 364:861
11. Owens C, Bui J, Knuttinen M, Gaba R et al (2010) Pulmonary embolism from upper extremity deep vein thrombosis and the role of superior vena cava filters: a review of the literature. J Vasc Interv Radiol 21:779
12. Hirsh J, Cogo A, Lensing A et al (1993) Distribution of thrombosis in patients with symptomatic deep vein thrombosis. Implications for simplifying the diagnostic process with compression ultrasound. JAMA 153:2777–2780
13. Elliott CG (2000) The diagnostic approach to deep venous thrombosis: diagnostic tests for deep vein thrombosis. Semin Respir Crit Care Med 21:6
14. Lensing A, Jongbloets L, Koopman M et al (1994) Limitations of compression ultrasound for the detection of symptomless postoperative deep vein thrombosis. Lancet 343:1142–1144
15. Bleichrodt H, Quiggin J (1999) Life-cycle preferences over consumption and health: when is cost-effectiveness analysis equivalent to cost-benefit analysis? J Health Econ 18:681–708
16. Gold MR et al (1996) Cost-effectiveness in health and medicine. Oxford University Press, New York/Oxford, p 18
17. Black W (2000) A graphical representation of cost-effectiveness. Med Decis Making 10:212–214
18. Infusion Nurses Society (2006) Infusion nursing standard of practice. J Infus Nurs 29(suppl1):S1–S92
19. Nifong T, McDevitt T (2011) The effect of catheter to vein ratio on blood flow rates in a simulated model of peripherally inserted central venous catheters. Chest 140:48–53
20. Dawson R (2011) PICC Zone Insertion Method (ZIM): a systematic approach to determine the ideal insertion site for PICCs in the upper arm. J Assoc Vasc Access 16:156–165

Advantages, Disadvantages, and Indications of PICCs in Inpatients and Outpatients

5

Baudolino Mussa

Long-term central venous access is essential for managing patients with cancer, congenital malformations, and gastrointestinal malfunction, as well as for delivering medication and blood product therapy. Peripherally inserted central venous catheters (PICC) address all of these needs. Also, they offer a less invasive, safe and effective alternative to other conventional and central venous access devices.

There are many reasons why PICCs are commonly used both inside and outside the hospital. They can be easily inserted and are cost-effective and convenient. They provide prolonged access for administrating medications, which would be otherwise irritating for smaller peripheral blood vessels, or supply nutrition via the venous route to patients unable to tolerate oral feedings, or deliver life-support therapies to the critically ill or injured. While PICCs afford many benefits, physicians, nurses, and patients still need to be aware of the risks associated with indwelling PICCs so that complications can be minimized. And although the complication rates of PICC lines are low, the lowest for all centrally placed IV access devises, serious complications can occur. Selecting a venous access device according to disease and patient can minimize complications and obtain optimal outcomes.

In 1929, Werner Forssmann self-experimented with cardiac catheterization, demonstrating that central catheterization through the antecubital vein in the arm was indeed possible. Only years later would this concept become widely accepted, opening the way to the later development of PICCs. With advances in material design and the use of echography to guide catheter insertion, the use of PICCs has gained wider application also in home-based IV therapies (Figs. 5.1 and 5.2). In both clinical and home-health settings, PICCs have been shown to adequately and safely meet the needs of patients under short- or long-term therapy.

The annual market growth of PICCs worldwide is about 6 %, accounting for the largest share of all vascular access device sales. PICC use in hospital as in homecare

B. Mussa
Digestive, Colorectal and Oncological Surgery Unit,
University of Turin Medical School, Turin, Italy
e-mail: baudolino.mussa@unito.it

S. Sandrucci, B. Mussa (eds.), *Peripherally Inserted Central Venous Catheters*,
DOI 10.1007/978-88-470-5665-7_5, © Springer-Verlag Italia 2014

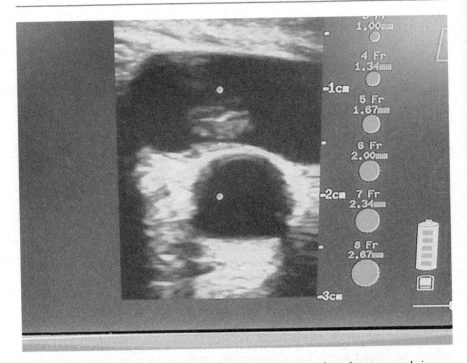

Fig. 5.1 Echographic aspect of an indwelling intravenous catheter through a transversal view

Fig. 5.2 Echographic aspect
of an indwelling intravenous
catheter through a
longitudinal view

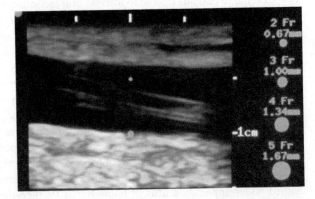

has expanded with the event of power injectable technology and new imaging technologies that can visualize correct catheter tip position. Central venous catheters (CVC) other than PICCs have been recognized as a reliable source of vascular access since the 1970s. PICCs became a popular central catheter in the early 1990s in adults and children. Because they can deliver drugs, liquids, or parenteral nutrition via a central vein, with the safety of a conventional peripheral venous access, PICCs can be considered as a "hybrid" between conventional peripheral venous access devices and CVCs.

Fig. 5.3 The exit site aspect of a 4-month implanted PICC

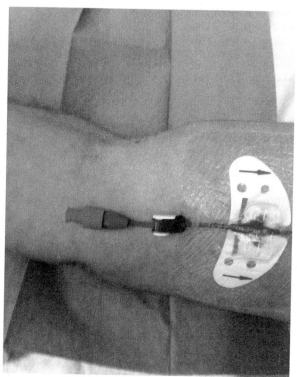

The advantages of PICCs are as follows:

Long-term venous access. A PICC is an ideal venous access device for patients with chronic diseases requiring long-term antibiotic or nutritional IV therapy. A conventional peripheral venous catheter is usually reinserted in a different site every 3–5 days, depending on the catheterization protocol adopted by a department. With proper care and maintenance, PICCs may last for up to 1 year, without changing the entry site and with minimal risk of complications (Fig. 5.3).

Low risk of infection. After prepping the site with chlorhexidine gluconate, a PICC is inserted using a sterile technique, and a disc impregnated with chlorhexidine gluconate is applied to the insertion site at each dressing change. In addition to ensuring that the dressing remains clean, dry, and intact, the use of chlorhexidine gluconate further reduces risk of infection. Additionally, a PICC is typically inserted into a vein in the upper arm, which is cleaner than other body areas such as the neck or the groin, where central lines are inserted. Lastly, because PICCs are long lasting, the risk of infection from changing insertion sites is eliminated.

Fewer skin punctures for blood draws. PICCs can be used to draw blood samples for diagnostic and clinical blood tests. The use of a PICC obviates the need for repeated skin punctures for blood sampling, minimizing the risk of infection and patient discomfort.

Fig. 5.4 A radiologically documented PICC catheter malposition in the axillary vein

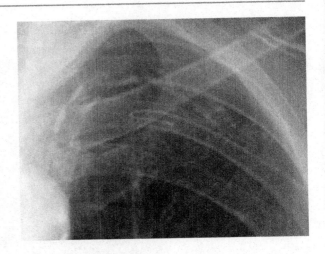

Early patient discharge. A PICC line can be adequately managed at home by healthcare agencies, caregivers, infusion centers, or other outpatient facilities. For example, patients requiring a 6-week regimen of IV antibiotics no longer need to be hospitalized to complete the course of treatment. Furthermore, the access line can remain in place for weeks or even up to 1 year, if necessary. The only other long-term IV access devices that meet this standard of long life and early discharge are implanted ports, which are invasive and considered a surgical procedure.

Versatility. PICC lines, by virtue of their multiple-lumen IV access, can be used to administer antibiotics, blood and blood products, anticancer drugs, intravenous fluids, and nutrients.

PICCs are not appropriate for every patient, however. Indications, contraindications, and potential complications need to be considered prior to placing a PICC line. Nor is the placement technique always easy and user friendly. Nurses and doctors must be familiar with the use of echography to identify the most suitable vein for long-term PICC placement and then, once identified, be able to insert a 20–21-gauge needle into a small vein (diameter, 3–6 mm), without injuring the median nerve which may pass near the vein precisely where it seemed the best site for line placement.

Reaching the right tip position poses particular challenges owing to anatomic obstructions or distortions, thrombosis, or abnormal course of the vein in the axillary or thoracic regions (Fig. 5.4). Obviously, a 40-cm catheter is less likely to reach the right position than a 20-cm catheter placed in the jugular vein.

Another issue is the flow rate of PICCs. Basically, a PICC is a long tube with a small internal diameter. The diameter of a PICC is ordinarily from 3 to 6 French (1–2 mm), whereas commonly used CVCs range in diameter from 5 to 12 French (1.7–4 mm). This difference in lumen size explains why PICCs have a lower volume flow rate than conventional catheters. Furthermore, Poiseuille's law states that the flow rate diminishes proportionally to the length of a tube and its diameter elevated to the power of four. Therefore, the flow rate in a 5-French PICC (length,

45 cm) will be 4.2 times less than that in a 7-French CVC (length, 20 cm). To increase volume flow through the line, power technology is applied to generate high pressure resistance (about 20 atm) which, in certain limited cases, can only be achieved using a contrast media infusor. This problem limits volume flow rates, especially in the delivery of high-density drugs. So blood, nutritional solutions, or certain drugs delivered via a PICC line require prolonged infusion or the use of an infusion pump.

Another problem with both valved and normal PICCs is that they require weekly irrigation to maintain catheter patency; either saline or heparinized solution is "pumped" through the PICC line.

Complications associated with PICC lines include the following:

- Air embolism. Air bubbles entering the blood vessel during PICC insertion may cause such symptoms as decreased blood pressure, lightheadedness, confusion, increased heart rate, anxiety, chest pain, or shortness of breath.
- Infections. Infections can develop either inside the vessel or around the insertion site where the catheter enters the vein. Symptoms of infection include fever, chills, tachycardia, fatigue, muscle aches, weakness, decreased blood pressure, redness, swelling or purulent drainage at the entry site, or elevated white blood cell count [5].
- Phlebitis of the vein at the insertion site. Symptoms of phlebitis include redness, tenderness around the entry site, palpable venous cord, or purulent drainage [7].
- Catheter malposition. Malposition can occur during PICC insertion or later due to catheter migration or changes in pressure inside the chest. After the catheter has been inserted, the position of its tip is confirmed by x-ray. Proper tip placement must be confirmed before the device can be used since a malpositioned catheter can cause serious complications. Securing the PICC is also essential to help prevent catheter dislodgment or migration. The catheter should not be secured to the site with sutures as these can cause infections at the site or catheter-related bloodstream infections.
- Thrombus formation. Any catheter inserted into the vascular system increases the risk of thrombus formation in either the vessel or the catheter [3].
- Difficult removal. Resistance may be encountered when removing the catheter and this may occur at any time during the procedure.
- Nerve injury or irritation. During catheter insertion, nearby nerves may be injured or become irritated, producing such symptoms as a shooting pain down the arm, numbness, tingling, pins and needles sensation, and limb weakness or paralysis.
- Leakage. Occasionally, leakage at the insertion site may occur. This may be caused by loss of elasticity of the skin at the access site, outward catheter migration, or catheter rupture (Fig. 5.5).
- Catheter breakage. Catheter damage occurs rarely and most often results from improper care. It may ensue from improper anchoring, the use of a syringe less than 10 ml, or applying excessive pressure when flushing the device (Fig. 5.6). If the catheter is placed in the elbow bend, breakage can also occur from repetitive motion, which should be avoided [4].

Fig. 5.5 Catheter rupture of the external portion of the device due to inappropriate nursing

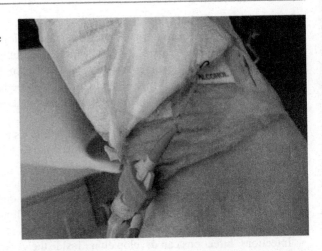

Fig. 5.6 Catheter damage as a result of an inappropriate flushing with a low-volume syringe

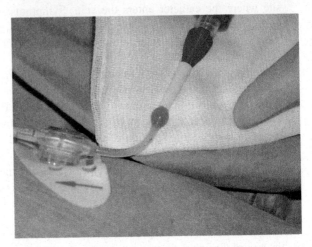

5.1   Safety Versus Problems of Total Parenteral Nutrition Therapy via PICC Lines

In some hospital settings, PICCs have become the preferred alternative over CVC lines inserted in the neck region for the administration of total parenteral nutrition therapy (TPN). This is related to three main factors: cost-effectiveness, ease of device insertion, and a significantly lower incidence of major complications.

Cost-effectiveness has become vital in this era of managed healthcare. As physician reimbursements for central line and PICC placement have steadily declined, specially trained and certified nursing teams have been delivering effective PICC placement services, beginning with insertion through to continuing care and education after the lines have been placed. The cost-effectiveness of such services has been demonstrated in numerous studies [2].

Ease of insertion compared to subclavian or internal jugular placement not only means greater cost-effectiveness in terms of the hours saved in trying to secure intravenous access but also making the procedure much more tolerable for patients. With PICC lines, the failure rate is significantly lower. There is significantly less tissue trauma and complication risks are substantially lower. In addition, the risk of infections is far lower with a PICC line in the upper arm than a central line inserted in the neck.

Major central venous complications include hemothorax, pneumothorax, cardiac tamponade, or blood vessel rupture, which are not typically present in PICC line placement. In addition, as compared with central catheterization, PICC tip migration is less frequent. Being at lower risk of complications, patients in a subacute setting, who are more likely to be conscious and eager to be discharged, experience much less anxiety. Monitoring PICC function is easy, an added advantage for their use in a domestic setting [6].

The only drawbacks to PICC versus central lines appear to be venous thrombophlebitis (10–30 %) [1] and line occlusion. These complications may require declotting an occluded line, which is highly successful and noninvasive, restarting lines at more frequent intervals or, in rare instances, conversion to central catheterization. In addition, PICCs may also be difficult to insert in certain patients, for example, those with very poor venous access, gross obesity, or exhaustion of viable veins due to repeated cannulation. Nonetheless, placement of other types of lines is subject to the same difficulties.

5.2   Why Are PICC Lines Used in Hospitalized Patients?

Venous access is an important part of treatment in every hospitalized patient. Because the peripheral venous network must be preserved to maintain a patient's future possibility of intravenous therapy, selecting the appropriate venous access is a critical step at the beginning of the therapeutic approach (Fig. 5.7). Timing, type, and morbidity are the key issues for the choice of the correct vascular access device. In this vision of healthcare, PICCs have become a major factor. PICC lines can be placed by nurses, thus reducing logistics costs; PICC lines are safer than CVCs in patients with thrombocytopenia or impaired coagulation and are easy to dress in patients with tracheostomy or other types of stoma. Finally, PICC lines have a long operating life. For every patient at risk of complications and eligible for IV therapy at home, a PICC may offer the right choice.

5.3   What Type of PICC Line?

For inpatients, open-tip power PICC lines are probably the best choice, as they have a limited cost and reliably allow to measure central venous pressure, take blood draws, and deliver contrast infusion. Open-tip PICC lines, to ensure a long operating life, require the use of good-quality neutral pressure "needle-free" connectors. The nurse's ability to use, dress, irrigate, and maintain this type of PICC is crucial. Another problem could be the occurrence of blood reflux at the end of a gravity

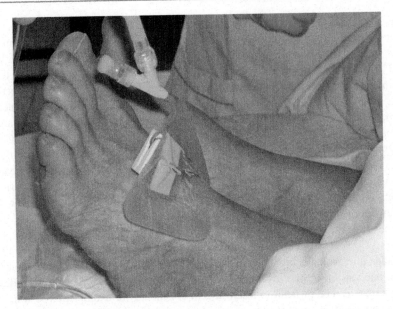

Fig. 5.7 An "extreme" approach to venous system requiring a radical change in the organization and management of therapeutic venous accesses

infusion that has not been correctly stopped. In such situations, because needle-free connectors cannot prevent against obstruction in a PICC due to blood reflux inside the line, open-tip PICCs must be employed with pumps, infusors, or other systems that can prevent reflux by positive pressure infusion.

5.4 Why Are PICC Lines Used in Homecare Patients?

PICC lines may be placed at the bedside in the patient's home without any additional risk. ECG-guided tip positioning minimizes the need for checking correct catheter placement by radiological control. PICC lines need weekly maintenance, which can be easily taught to the caregiver. Well-placed PICC lines are a safe way to deliver IV therapy and take blood draws. The main drawback of home PICC lines is that they make taking a shower or bath difficult for the patient. Recognizing this problem, industries are developing waterproof dressings for this purpose. A polyurethane self-adhesive dressing should always be used to protect the PICC exit site from water exposure.

5.5 What Type of PICC Line?

In homecare, one of the major risks is damage to the external part of a PICC line and occlusion due to an incorrectly stopped infusion: valved PICCs can adequately meet most homecare needs. Proximal and distal valves close the PICC when the pressure is too low to open them. So, if a PICC line is damaged or disconnected, or at the end of an infusion, the low inflow pressure closes the valve, thus preventing backflow and occlusion. Thanks to their safety and ease of use, valved PICCs are preferred in the homecare setting.

References

1. Periard D, Monney P, Waeber G, Zurkinden C, Mazzolai L, Hayoz D, Doenz F, Zanetti G, Wasserfallen JB, Denys A (2008) Randomized controlled trial of peripherally inserted central catheters vs. peripheral catheters for middle duration in-hospital intravenous therapy. J Thromb Haemost 6(8):1281–1288
2. Robinson MK, Mogensen KM, Grudinskas GF, Kohler S, Jacobs DO (2005) Improved care and reduced costs for patients requiring peripherally inserted central catheters: the role of bedside ultrasound and a dedicated team. J Parenter Enteral Nutr 29(5):374–379
3. Lobo BL, Vaidean G, Broyles J, Reaves AB, Shorr RI (2009) Risk of venous thromboembolism in hospitalized patients with peripherally inserted central catheters. J Hosp Med 4(7):417–422
4. Bowers L, Speroni KG, Jones LA, Atherton M (2009) Comparison of occlusion rates by flushing solutions for peripherally inserted central catheters with positive pressure Luer activated devices. J Infus Nurs 31(1):22–27
5. Ajenjo MC, Morley JC, Russo AJ, McMullen KM, Robinson C, Williams RC, Warren DK (2011) Peripherally inserted central venous catheter–associated bloodstream infections in hospitalized adult patients. Infect Control Hosp Epidemiol 32(2):85–90
6. Stokowski G, Steele D, Wilson D (2009) The use of ultrasound to improve practice and reduce complication rates in peripherally inserted central catheter insertions: final report of investigation. J Infus Nurs 32(3):145–155
7. Marnejon T, Angelo D, Abu Abdou A, Gemmel D (2012) Risk factors for upper extremity venous thrombosis associated with peripherally inserted central venous catheters. J Vasc Access 13(2):231–238

Ultrasound Anatomy of Peripheral Veins and Ultrasound-Guided Venipuncture

6

Nancy L. Moureau

As the specialty art and practice of placing intravenous devices continues to evolve, ultrasound provides a means to identify and assess veins as well as guide the insertion of access devices for catheter placement, resulting in greater success and patient safety. The identification of peripheral veins can be challenging due to skin color, vein size, depth, and distribution. Ultrasound is especially helpful in vein identification and needle guidance with peripherally inserted central catheters (PICCs). The insertion of peripheral venous access devices into the small veins of the arm is a skill requiring fine motor movement is aided by ultrasound. The insertion of these devices is primarily done in the upper extremities for peripherally inserted central catheters (PICCs). Veins of the lower extremities may be used in pediatric patients or critically ill adults requiring femoral access. This chapter focuses on ultrasound-guided insertion in the upper arm and offers a brief overview of the identification of the veins specific to the upper arm and placement of PICCs; assessment of the vasculature, and a step-by-step process for venipuncture with ultrasound.

6.1 Anatomy and Identification of Veins Using Ultrasound

Since the vast majority of peripheral vascular access devices are inserted in veins of the upper extremities, descriptions of vein characteristics will focus on the basilic, brachial, and cephalic veins (see Fig. 6.1).

Successful ultrasound-guided venipuncture is based, in part, on the ability to locate a vein, determine the depth, select the most appropriate needle length and catheter size for that vein, and access and then advance the catheter into the vein. This applies to the insertion of peripherally inserted central catheters (PICCs),

N.L. Moureau, BSN, RN, CRNI, CPUI, VA-BC
Department of Vascular Access, PICC Excellence, Inc., 1905 Whippoorwill Trail, Hartwell, GA 30643, USA

Greenville Memorial System University Medical Center, Greenville, SC, USA
e-mail: nancy@piccexcellence.com

S. Sandrucci, B. Mussa (eds.), *Peripherally Inserted Central Venous Catheters*,
DOI 10.1007/978-88-470-5665-7_6, © Springer-Verlag Italia 2014

Fig. 6.1 Peripheral veins
(Courtesy of PICC
Excellence Inc.)

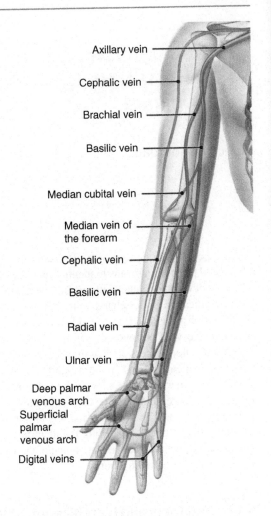

Axillary vein

Cephalic vein

Brachial vein

Basilic vein

Median cubital vein

Median vein of
the forearm

Cephalic vein

Basilic vein

Radial vein

Ulnar vein

Deep palmar
venous arch
Superficial
palmar
venous arch

Digital veins

midlines, and ultrasound-guided peripheral catheters. Peripheral veins of the arm have depths that vary from very superficial to deeper, 5.0 cm with obese patients. Veins most suitable for venous access range from 0.25 to 2 cm. Vein size without the aid of a tourniquet, as measured by diameter, may be as small as 1–2 mm in the lower arm and up to 16 mm in the upper arm. Veins selected for use with venous access are ideally three times the diameter size of the selected catheter (e.g., a 4-French or 18-gauge catheter requires a 4 mm or larger vein), allowing for adequate blood flow around the catheter, providing protection to the vein walls from the catheter, and also providing ample dilution of the infusate with the blood as it passes from the catheter into the vein [1–3].

The identification of veins of the arm with ultrasound is facilitated by beginning at the antecubital fossa where the veins are most superficial. The first structures which may be visible to the eye are the median or cubital veins directly at the center of the antecubital fossa. Visualizing deeper with ultrasound, look for the brachial artery and brachial veins located near the center of the arm and the basilic vein located along the medial aspect. The basilic vein is the most commonly used vein for PICC placement. The cephalic vein is present on the lateral side of the arm and tends to be small with a more tortuous path. Direct access at the antecubital fossa is generally discouraged due to the amount of joint movement associated with this location. Movement of a catheter in and out of an insertion site contributes to the development of phlebitis and other complications. Finding a stable location at least 4 cm or more above the antecubital fossa provides stability and reduces movement.

The veins of the upper arm are used for placement of peripherally inserted central catheters (PICCs) and midlines. Three main vessels are present in the upper arm: basilic, brachial, and cephalic veins.

6.2   Basilic

The first vein of choice for a PICC placement is the basilic vein running along the medial side of the arm. This vein is the largest and straightest vein in the arm, averaging 6–8 mm in diameter at the antecubital region. At its upper limit where the basilic and brachial veins join the axillary vein, the basilic vein may reach 10–14 mm in diameter. The basilic vein is present at varying depths from 0.5 to 5 cm. Since it is not generally accompanied by an artery or a nerve, access into the basilic vein has a lower risk of complications than with the brachial veins. Additionally, a right-sided basilic access is preferred over the left due to the increase in complications associated with left-sided insertions. Left-sided insertions have a greater distance and more acute angle as the catheter exits the innominate/brachiocephalic vein and enters the superior vena cava.

6.3   Brachial Vein(s)

The brachial vein(s), located in the brachial bundle, is also used for PICC placement but carries greater risk due to the depth and close proximity to the brachial artery and nerve bundle. The two brachial veins, known as a venae comitantes, Latin for accompanying veins, are encased in a thin sheath with the brachial artery and median nerve forming the brachial bundle. The brachial bundle is easy to detect as it has a configuration that looks like Mickey Mouse (see Fig. 6.2).

The brachial bundle becomes most apparent above the antecubital fossa. The first rule of ultrasound is to locate arteries and nerves in the insertion area prior to needle access. In the case of an upper arm insertion, the brachial artery and the median nerve need to be identified prior to upper arm access. In Fig. 6.2, note the configuration of the brachial bundle, two veins on either side, and in this image, the median nerve is directly on top of the brachial artery. The median nerve is a significantly large structure that should always be identified and avoided. To visualize the median nerve, look above or to the side of the brachial artery and vein for a circular

Fig. 6.2 Brachial bundle
with median nerve, and
basilic vein (Courtesy of
PICC Excellence Inc.)

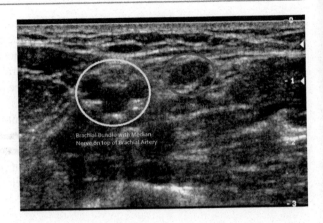

grouping or cluster, dark with light borders, sometimes appearing as a noncompressible vein. Needle penetration of the median nerve results in a severe electrical
shooting pain, paresthesia, numbness, and aching and, with more significant nerve
contact, can cause muscle contraction. Removing the needle is the standard of practice when symptoms of nerve impingement occur. Use ultrasound to clearly note the
location of the nerve prior to beginning a second access attempt. The best approach
to accessing a brachial vein while avoiding the median nerve may be from the side,
a more lateral approach as opposed to a center, straight down access. The brachial
vein pair advances up the arm deep within the muscle and joins with the basilic or
directly into the axillary vein.

6.4   Cephalic Vein

The cephalic vein is usually visible on the lateral aspect of the arm. Due to its small
size, approximately 6 mm in diameter at the antecubital fossa in an average adult,
it is less desirable than the brachial or basilic veins for PICC insertion. Typically
the cephalic has many tributaries vein junction, high on the shoulder getting smaller
as it travels down the arm. Typically, it has many tributaries and a tortuous path
through its course in the arm. Secondary to its small size and convoluted path,
blood flow around an indwelling catheter may be compromised, resulting in phlebitis and vein damage post insertion. Cephalic vein access should be avoided if
possible.

Evaluation of veins to select the best location and device for insertion should
incorporate the RACEVA (rapid central vein assessment) method. This system was
designated by Pittiruti and associates as a method of vein assessment evaluating the
internal jugular, subclavian, brachiocephalic, axillary, basilic, and brachial veins as
all possible options. Using ultrasound allows you to select the vein with the safest
approach, best chance of success and lowest overall risk to the patient [4].

6.5   Vein Assessment

Prior to 1999, venous assessment incorporated visual assessment and palpation, known as a "blind approach," with landmarks to guide the inserter. With ultrasound readily available in all hospitals, ultrasound-guided insertions have become the standard of practice for insertion of all central venous catheters as a means to ensure safety for patients. Ultrasound-guided insertions involve more than just placing the probe, finding the round black vein, and inserting the needle. Skilled clinicians take the time to perform a thorough assessment, evaluating veins above and below an intended site, alternate veins, and looking at characteristics of healthy versus damaged veins. Upon completion of the assessment, the clinician can progress with the insertion with security, knowing which vein is the best choice and is most likely to result in success.

Proceeding with an ultrasound assessment of the peripheral veins of the arm depends in part on the type of device requested for insertion. Placement of a PICC involves different areas of veins versus those used for a shorter peripheral catheter. PICCs focus on the veins of the upper arm and specifically on the middle section of the upper arm for best results [5]. Regardless of the vein chosen, certain vein features are assessed.

Prior to beginning the scan of the arm, mentally review each of the steps to lead you to a successful evaluation of the veins of the patient's arm.

- Have the patient positioned comfortably with the arm abducted away from the body in a comfortable position to prevent muscle contraction.
- Position yourself with respect to the patient and the ultrasound device so you are comfortable with your weight evenly balanced.
- Check room lighting.
- Apply gel liberally to probe head for best visualization.
- Confirm hand position on the probe with the thumb on one side of probe and the index and middle fingers on the opposite side of the probe. The remaining fingers and lateral aspect of hand form the base and rest on the patient's arm.
- Confirm screen/probe orientation by lifting the right side of the probe off the skin and looking for image loss on the right side of the screen.

Characteristics evaluated during a vein assessment to determine vessel health and to select the best vein for venipuncture include:

- Vessel size
- Vessel location and path
- Vessel health
- Flow characteristics

A vessel should be of adequate size to support the catheter required for the delivery of medications. The recommended vessel size is three times that of the catheter. In other words, the catheter should not take up more than 1/3 of the diameter of the vessel lumen [3]. This allows for adequate blood flow around the catheter, reducing the risk of stasis, thrombosis, phlebitis, and other complications. Vessels should be assessed in their native state, without a tourniquet, to determine actual vessel size. Use the measuring device or sized images available on the ultrasound unit to measure exact lumen size; then compare this to the size of the catheter required to ensure the vein is large enough to accommodate the catheter.

During your initial assessment, evaluate the general path of a vessel. If a vessel has collaterals, areas of narrowing/stenosis, or makes unexpected dips, twists, and turns along its way up the arm and toward the heart, it may be difficult to advance a catheter through this vein. These characteristics may also represent vein damage. Collaterals may result in loops or dead ends. If the vessel is too tortuous, another vessel may need to be selected to provide for adequate flow and advancement of the catheter. Ultrasound makes it possible to follow the chosen vein all the way up to the shoulder and beyond to verify a patent pathway prior to insertion.

As you follow the vessel toward the heart with the ultrasound probe, consider the health of the vessel. Vessels should increase in size as they advance toward the heart. The veins should have a symmetrical appearance and the vessel walls should appear smooth. Observe for irregularities in vessel size, vessel shape, lumen size, and vessel wall thickness. Check for compressibility. Veins should easily compress with light to moderate pressure, pressing flat without any sign of scar tissue or thrombosis. Compression is one of the easiest and most reliable methods to check a vein for thrombosis. If a vein does not compress or collapse with light to moderate pressure or compresses in a lopsided way, thrombosis may be present in the vein. Turn the probe to view the vein longitudinally. By viewing the vein walls in a longer view you can effectively assess for abnormailities or vein problems.

Flow characteristics within the vessel may be assessed using the color pulse Doppler (CPD) available on most ultrasound units. CPD cannot be used to calculate an exact flow rate; however, it can be used to confirm the presence of flow and to get a general feel of flow volume. This is useful for veins where thrombosis is suspected, when observing the path of the vein, or when determining if a vessel is a vein or an artery. Using CPD, angle the beam off ninety degrees and watch for the vessel to "light up." Bright red to gold color shifts are visible on the ultrasound screen based on the number of red blood cells passing beneath the probe, demonstrating active flow. If the vessel is an artery, you will see pulsatile flow light up on the screen with each heartbeat. Changes in flow channels represent vein wall abnormalities like partial occlusion or prior recannulation of an older thrombus.

6.6   Systematic Assessment

1. Position the probe at the antecubital fossa to begin your scan. Locate the brachial bundle then move medial to locate the basilic vein. Scan up the arm for PICC or midline vein assessment, down for peripheral catheters.
2. Begin narrowing your choices looking for veins 0–2 cm in depth, 1 cm or less being ideal. Select the vein of choice for your device and mark the area. Optimal location for a PICC is in the center of the upper arm (Dawson, 2011).
3. Compress the vein with tourniquet pressure in place. Verify even compression and vessel closure without pulsation.

4. Locate arteries. Locate the brachial artery and median nerve in the brachial bundle.
5. Follow the path of your chosen vein up the arm to the shoulder looking for areas of narrowing, irregular compression, signs of thrombosis, or collateral veins.
6. Go beyond the shoulder and view the axillary vein and artery. Ask the patient about filters, surgery, or anything that might hamper your catheter advancement.
7. Go back to the marked vein and proceed down the arm. Look for areas of thrombosis that may propagate up to your chosen site.
8. Once you have confirmed the health and viability of the vein, go back to your mark and measure the diameter without a tourniquet in place. Compare your diameter with the catheter size to ensure more than 2/3 of the vein is left open for blood flow.
9. Proceed with setup and insertion.

6.7 Step by Step Ultrasound-Guided Needle Access for PICC

1. Wash hands and apply clean gloves as appropriate.
2. Apply a tourniquet and assess the veins of the arm with ultrasound.
3. Mark chosen vein location; apply gel to ultrasound probe head and set on stand.
4. Measure from marked vein to superior vena cava for estimated PICC length.
5. Collect and position supplies.
6. Disinfect skin with alcoholic chlorhexidine.
7. Apply tourniquet.
8. Prepare sterile field and maximum sterile barriers for PICC insertion.
9. Clean skin again and drape patient (full body drape for PICCs).
10. Cover ultrasound probe in a sterile fashion per protocol.
11. Apply sterile gel to covered probe; view selected vein at mark.
12. Administer anesthetic as needed.
13. For needle guide: Place the needle in guide for designated vein depth. Insert the needle through the skin. Visualize the path of the needle on ultrasound view screen. Observe the needle touching the top of vein wall and penetrating the vein (see Fig. 6.3). Verify blood return.
14. For free-hand insertion: Insert the needle close to the midpoint of probe face leaning probe back, away from the needle to view the insertion. As you advance the needle, straighten the probe to perpendicular and follow the point of the needle. Slide the probe as needed to keep advancing, keeping the point of the needle in view. Observe the needle touching the vein wall and penetrating the vein. Verify blood return.
15. Advance wire through the needle. Remove the needle. Follow the PICC procedure.

Ultrasound can be used to verify the needle or wire in the vein by using a longitudinal or sagittal view of the vein (see Fig. 6.4). Following the insertion of the PICC, ultrasound can also be used to rule out the placement of the catheter in the

Fig. 6.3 Needle penetrating
the vein (Courtesy of PICC
Excellence Inc.)

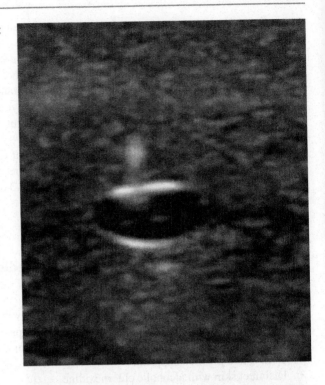

Fig. 6.4 Longitudinal view
of the vein and needle
(Courtesy of PICC
Excellence Inc.)

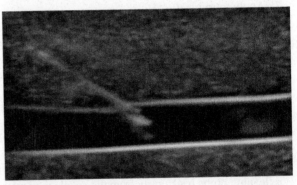

internal jugular vein. Place the ultrasound probe at the base of the neck and flush the
catheter briskly looking for bubbles and movement in the vein.

6.8   Tracking the Needle on the Ultrasound Screen

The needle produces two distinct ultrasound images as it passes through the arm.
The first is produced by the tip or echogenic portion of the shaft and the second is
produced by the smooth part of the shaft. It is imperative that you learn to track the

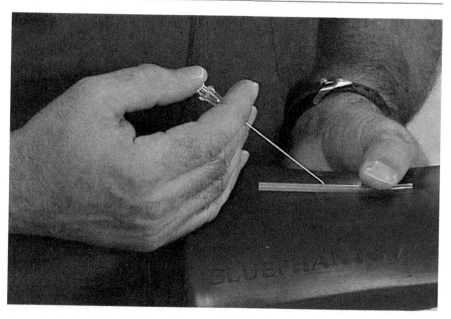

Fig. 6.5 Ultrasound practice pad (Courtesy of PICC Excellence Inc.)

tip of the needle and not the needle shaft for successful vein access. Because the needle shaft is smooth and not echogenic, it does not appear on the screen; rather, it produces movement of the surrounding tissue as it travels toward the vein. This is similar to water movement as a boat moves through causing waves known as a wake. While the general idea of the needle path is helpful to understand, it does not necessarily indicate the position of the needle tip. If a vein is curved slightly and the wake is seen heading toward the vein, the tip may be just far enough off track to miss the vein entirely. Practice watching the tip of the needle using an ultrasound phantom vein pad (or turkey breasts with inserted tubes to simulate veins) over and over until you can clearly see the difference between the tip and the wake (Fig. 6.5). Then, consistently track the tip through 12 or more practice accesses.

To ensure needle visualization under the probe face, check the depth to the top edge of the vein on the ultrasound screen and then place the needle back from the probe that same distance. For example, if the vein is 1 cm deep, then insert the needle approximately 1 cm back from the center of the probe. As the needle moves down to the vein, it will become visible on the ultrasound screen at a 1 cm depth on top of the vein.

The rough surface of the needle bevel and the echogenic portion of the shaft near the tip of the needle both produce a bright white image on the screen. This bright white image should be kept in view on the ultrasound screen throughout the entire insertion procedure from the time the needle penetrates the skin until it enters into the vein. Watch this image push down on the vein and enter the lumen. Once the needle enters the lumen of the vein, look for blood return at the hub of the needle. If there is no blood, perhaps the vein is just compressed and not yet pierced, so continue slowly. If the lower vein wall is moving, the needle may have gone through the lower vein wall and needs to be withdrawn slowly until blood return is established. Make small adjustments of just a few millimeters in distance each time you move the needle. If you see the needle inside the vein but adjacent to the wall and you do not have a blood return, try rotating the needle 90° as the bevel may be up against the vessel wall. Ultrasound increases insertion safety by guiding single-wall penetration rather than accidental double-wall puncture that allows leakage of blood into the tissues causing hematoma formation.

Conclusion

Ultrasound-guided PICC access aids the clinician in vein identification, assessment, and insertion in many ways that promote the highest level of safety for patients. Not only does the use of ultrasound increase the clinician's success on insertion, after competency has been achieved, but it also reduces the risk of many complications including infection. The time to successful insertion is decreased, trauma and complications are reduced, and stress to patients is minimized. There is no reason, in this day and age, not to use ultrasound during the insertion of central venous catheters. Overall, the application of ultrasound technology to all peripheral venous accesses is to the advantage of the patient, the clinician, and the facility.

References

1. Nifong TP, McDevitt TJ (2011) The effect of catheter to vein ratio on blood flow rates in a simulated model of peripherally inserted central catheters. Chest 140:48–53
2. Moureau NL, Trick N, Nifong T, Perry C, Kelley C, Carrico R, Leavitt M, Gordon SM, Wallace J, Harvill M, Biggar C, Doll M, Papke L, Benton L, Phelan DA (2012) Vessel health and preservation (Part 1): a new evidence-based approach to vascular access selection and management. J Vasc Access 13(3):351–356
3. Moureau Nancy L, King Kathy (2007) Advanced Ultrasound Assessment. PICC Excellence Inc http://www.piccexcellence.com/account_center/Adv_Ultrsnd/class_demo/?phpMyAdmin =5d8c508a98ebt6b307419&phpMyAdmin=5ebc509952e6t1f17bac0&phpMyAdmin=5H2XZ VWotZ%2ChqdfD7JnIqkuOmi5. Accessed 14 Oct 2013
4. Pittiruti M (2012) RaCeVA: a guide for a rational choice of the most appropriate vein for central venous catheterization 26th annual Association of Vascular Access (AVA)l Conference, San Antonio
5. Dawson RB (2011) PICC zone insertion method (zim): a systematic approach to determine the ideal insertion site for PICCs in the upper arm. JAVA 16(3):156–165

Evaluation Techniques of the PICC Tip Placement

7

Antonio La Greca

7.1 Introduction

Correct tip position of a peripherally inserted central venous catheter (PICC), as well as for any kind of central venous catheter, is of paramount importance in order to ensure good catheter performances and to prevent severe complications such as venous thrombosis or vessel/heart perforation. Unfortunately, PICCs are prone to high rates (up to 32 %) of primary malposition [1], if placed without any intraoperative method of tip control, due to their pronounced flexibility and the long route they must go through to reach the atriocaval junction.

Primary tip malposition not only exposes the patient to a wide range of infusion-related complications but also increases the average cost of the procedure, especially in high-volume centers, as it requires at least an over-guidewire replacement, in most cases a completely new venipuncture.

7.2 Optimal Tip Location and Classification of Primary Malpositions

Even though a widespread agreement regarding the correct position for the tip of a central venous catheter (CVC) does not exist yet [2], we assume, according to most US and European experts and guidelines, that the correct position is anywhere between the lower third of the superior vena cava and the upper region of the right atrium, regardless of the type of technique used (surgical cutdown, percutaneous puncture) and of the choice of the vein (brachial, basilic, internal jugular, subclavian, external jugular, etc.). The junction between the superior vena cava and the right atrium is considered the

A. La Greca
Department of Surgical Sciences, "A. Gemelli" Hospital – Catholic University,
Largo Agostino Gemelli 8, Rome 00168, Italy
e-mail: antonio.lagreca@rm.unicatt.it

S. Sandrucci, B. Mussa (eds.), *Peripherally Inserted Central Venous Catheters*,
DOI 10.1007/978-88-470-5665-7_7, © Springer-Verlag Italia 2014

optimal site for the tip of infusion devices [3–6], as it allows drug delivery in a high-blood-flow environment, thus avoiding chemical irritation of endothelium, and the alignment of the catheter with the main axis of the vessel, thus preventing mechanical irritation of endothelium. In this way, the two most important etiological factors for venous thrombosis and catheter malfunction are eliminated [7–9].

Primary malposition occurs when the implantation procedure fails to place the tip of the catheter in the abovementioned location (close to the atriocaval junction), while "secondary malposition" identifies tip migration from the correct location to a wrong one days/weeks/months after a successful procedure. This chapter is mainly focused on prevention of primary malposition, but some issues may apply to secondary malposition as well.

Primary malpositions may be classified as follows [10]:

1. "High" malposition – that is the catheter tip located in the ipsilateral internal jugular/subclavian vein, typically observed after the insertion of the catheter in the subclavian or internal jugular vein, due to the impaired progression into the brachiocephalic trunk.
2. "Low" malposition – that is the catheter tip located in the contralateral brachiocephalic/jugular/subclavian due to the catheter failing to enter the superior vena cava.
3. "Short" catheter – that is the catheter tip located in the middle third or upper third of the superior vena cava. Short catheters inserted from the left side of the patient carry a higher risk of vessel damage due to both chemical and mechanical endothelial irritation and are frequently associated with the occurrence of "secondary malposition" or "tip migration" [7, 11].
4. "Long" catheter – that is the catheter tip located in the middle third or lower third of the right atrium, or in the right ventricle, or in the inferior vena cava (suprarenal inferior vena cava if approaching from the femoral vein).
5. Catheter tip in secondary or anomalous vessels (azygos, hemiazygos, internal mammary vein, etc.) – quite rare.

Malposition types 1, 2, 3, and 5 are at high risk for catheter malfunction and venous thrombosis [7, 8], while type 4 exposes the patient to a high risk of arrhythmias, heart cavity lesions/perforation, tricuspid valve dysfunction or lesions, and thrombosis [9, 12].

7.3 "Predictive" Methods to Prevent Primary Malpositions

A number of "tips" are currently used to prevent errors in catheter length and direction.

7.3.1 Catheter Length

The operator may use a combination of pre- and intraoperative criteria that can predict the expected final length of the catheter and/or help directing the catheter in the right direction.

"Predictive" methods that can estimate the expected catheter length are:

- Topographical anatomy landmarks: commonly, the atriocaval junction is assumed to be in correspondence of the right parasternal line at the third intercostal space. The expected catheter length can be calculated measuring on the patient's surface the distance from the selected venipuncture site to the abovementioned landmark.
- Algorithms based on anthropometric data of the patient:
  - Height in adults for catheters placed via cervicothoracic route, according to the different venipuncture approaches:
    - Subclavian vein by subclavear medial approach or IJV by posterosuperior approach [13]
    - Internal jugular vein by posteroinferior approach (S. Sandrucci, Lecture, Annual Master Course on Central Venous Access, Catholic University, Rome 2004)
    - Axillary vein by subclavear lateral ultrasound-guided approach (A. La Greca, Lecture, Annual Master Course on Central Venous Access, Catholic University, Rome 2013)
  - Weight/height in infants [14–17] for catheters placed via cervicothoracic approach.
  - For PICC lines, multiple anthropometric formulas are available [18]. A simple option could be measuring the distance from the selected venipuncture site to the sternoclavicular notch, and then add the result to a standard value of 10 cm if the catheter comes from the right arm and of 15 cm if it comes from the left arm (Caillouet B, MD Anderson Cancer Center, Implementation of Evidence-based Guide to Estimate PICC Length for Upper Arm Insertions for Placement into Distal Superior Vena Cava. Poster Presentation at Intravenous Nurses Society, Nashville, Tennessee, USA, May 2009).

These methods, although useful and included in the insertion protocols of most working groups, remain merely predictive of the expected catheter length in a specific patient and do not give any information about the actual tip location. In other words, even if the operator is able to exactly estimate the correct length of the catheter, that is, 35 cm, he or she will never know where actually the 35 cm of intravascular catheter have gone, unless he performs some kind of diagnostic procedure to locate the tip.

7.3.2 Catheter Direction

Several methods may help the operator to direct the catheter along the correct route (i.e., towards the superior vena cava):

- Routine adoption of CVC insertion techniques with low risk of malposition, for example, ultrasound-guided venipuncture by a supraclavicular approach, preferably on the right side. This option is obviously not suitable for PICCs.
- Rely on easy progression of a J guidewire, assuming that an early stop may be the expression of the J tip entering a tributary vein and advancing distally, being

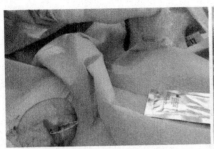 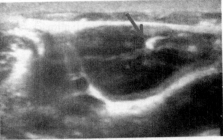

Fig. 7.1 Detection of primary malposition in the homolateral internal jugular vein (*arrow*) by ultrasound neck scanning during peripherally inserted central venous catheter (PICC) insertion

thus unable to go farther because of the narrowing vein lumen. This option is not suitable for PICCs because:

- In most cases, they are inserted by means of a modified Seldinger technique ("catheter through introducer"), meaning that the wire is not within the vessel while the catheter is advanced through the introducer.
- Even if a "direct" Seldinger technique is chosen, a soft and straight-tipped wire is commonly used in order to let it go through the peripheral access veins, narrower than the "central" ones.

• Threading the guidewire (if a "direct" Seldinger technique is chosen) or the catheter deeper than the expected length, until arrhythmias occur. Obviously, such a method is significantly dangerous for the patient and should be abandoned; nonetheless, it has been described and in use for years.

• Intra-procedural use of ultrasound for ruling out misdirection of the catheter. This procedure, based on the concept of the "negative assessment," is commonly performed exploring the great SVC tributary vessels (IJV, axillary, and brachiocephalic veins bilaterally) by the same US linear probe used during the venipuncture to identify whether the catheter (or the guidewire if a direct Seldinger technique is used) has entered the wrong vessel (Fig. 7.1). Eventually, the IVC can be explored as well using a convex medium-frequency probe. Even if some types of malposition cannot be ruled out, such as catheters "too short" in the SVC, "too long" deep in the right atrium, or misplaced in unexplorable veins (i.e., azygos, internal mammary and others), this method can help the operator avoid the most common malpositions and achieve a good rate of correct tip placement at first attempt [19].

These methods do not have any value in determining the final direction of the catheter, its length, or the actual position of the tip: at the end of the procedure, the catheter may still be in a SVC tributary vein or with the tip too high (upper third of the superior vena cava) or too low (right atrium, inferior vena cava, ventricle). Both length and direction predictive methods still need something else to ensure that the tip has actually reached the atriocaval junction.

Fig. 7.2 The tracheal carina as a reference radiologic landmark to define the position of the tip of a central catheter in relation to the atriocaval junction: *a*=distance of the tip from the carina; *b*=reference line marking the level of the tip on the X-ray film; *arrow*=tip of the venous catheter

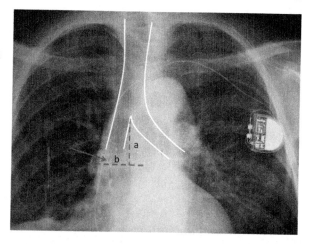

7.4   Diagnostics of Tip Location: How to Rule Out Primary Malposition

Checking catheter tip position may be performed during the procedure, after the procedure, or both.

7.4.1   Post-procedural Diagnosis of Tip Position

Traditionally, a standard single-view anteroposterior chest X-ray film has been considered the gold standard method not only for ruling out gross primary malposition but even to ascertain with a sufficient accuracy the exact position of the tip [20]. On a standard anteroposterior X-ray film, tip position is assessed using specific radiologic landmarks of the atriocaval junction. Among the different landmarks, the tracheal carina has been recently regarded as the most effective one, as it lies in the same plane of the cardiovascular mediastinum (thus avoiding misinterpretations due to parallax phenomenons), with precise and constant relationships with the right atrium, and allows location of the different anatomical subregions of the atriocaval junction [21, 22] (Fig. 7.2):

- SVC-RA junction: 3 cm under the tracheal carina
- Lower third of the SVC: under the carina but within the first 3 distal cm
- Upper third of the RA: from 3 to 5 cm under the carina

Considering the low cost and the diagnostic results of chest X-ray as compared to more refined but more expensive (and in some cases invasive) imaging techniques, such as MR and CT scan, this method is the most cost-effective among the post-procedural ones.

On the other hand, it is obvious that a post-procedural diagnosis of malposition requires the repositioning of the venous access: a further procedure which implies logistical problems and significant costs.

7.4.2 Intra-procedural Diagnosis of Tip Location

Checking the position of the tip of the catheter during the procedure is preferable to a post-procedural control [5]. During catheter insertion, the correct position of the catheter tip can be checked by different methods:

- Use of specific navigation ("tracking") devices, mainly adopting electromagnetic technology
- Intraoperative fluoroscopy and/or intraoperative control radiography
- Standard transthoracic echocardiography
- Transesophageal echocardiography
- The electrocardiographic method (intracavitary eKG)
- Combination methods

7.4.2.1 Navigation Methods

Navigation systems are mainly based on electromagnetic tracking of the catheter tip. Usually, the catheter is assembled with a specific magnetic stylet, which can be located by some kind of magnetic sensor placed on the patient's chest surface, either fixed on the chest wall or handheld by the operator. This allows the tip to be followed during its progression into the venous system by means of a virtual image on a specific screen or visual/acoustic alerts on the sensor placed on the chest surface or both (Fig. 7.3). At least three devices are available on the market (Navigator, by Viasys/Corpak; Sherlock, by Bard Access Systems Inc.; Cath-Finder, by Pharmacia Deltec), sharing the same functioning principles but with different technical issues deserving a specific dissertation which is not in the scope of this chapter.

Purely navigation systems are effective in preventing misdirection of the catheter ("gross" primary malposition) [1], but the exact tip position remains uncertain, as it is localized over a surface thoracic landmark that may be unreliable due to the variable relationships between the atriocaval junction and chest wall bones. Moreover, an anteroposterior misdirection of the catheter (i.e., azygos vein or internal mammary), even if rare, cannot be excluded. Thus, a post-procedural chest X-ray is still needed to finally locate the tip and obtain a documentation [23].

Recently, combination methods, assembling navigation and intracavitary EKG-based tip location technologies together in a single device, have also been tested in clinical trials and will be briefly described later on.

7.4.2.2 Fluoroscopy

Fluoroscopy is the most traditional and well-known intra-procedural method to determine the position of the tip of a central venous catheter, and thus its specific characteristics will not be discussed here. Its application to PICC insertion encounters several problems:

- Costs of the method are as high as 500–1,000 € per hour or procedure, depending on the local logistics.
- In high-volume centers (>500 line insertion per year), radiation protection issues for operators may be challenging and expensive.
- The use of fluoroscopy needs a dedicated shielded environment against ionizing radiations and is thus not applicable to bedside procedures in the wards (a widespread setting for PICC insertion) and not easy to arrange for outpatient (DH/ambulatory) procedures.

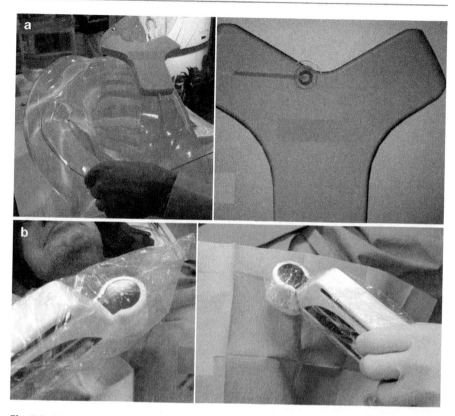

Fig. 7.3 Electromagnetic tracking. (**a**) Example of electromagnetic sensor fixed on the chest wall; note the separated screen showing the direction of the catheter; (**b**) example of handheld electromagnetic sensor detecting the tip of the catheter/stylet and showing the direction of the catheter

- Nurses are not homogeneously allowed and/or trained to use ionizing radiation for diagnostic purposes worldwide [20].
- The reliability of radiologic landmarks shares the same limits with plain chest X-ray.
- A general trend in increasing patients' safety by reducing their radiation exposure is taking place in the international health system, as encouraged by the recent AHRQ recommendations on this topic [24].

Despite these problems, fluoroscopy still represents a reference method for tip location due to its high accuracy, its apparently intuitive anatomical feedback, and the chance it offers to rule out pleural complications at the same time.

7.4.2.3 Ultrasound for Tip Location

Ultrasound can be used not only for the "negative assessment" of a catheter misdirection, as previously described, but even to directly or indirectly identify the catheter tip within the right atrium and/or in the lower part of the SVC (so-called positive assessment).

Different techniques for US-based identification of the tip have been described:
- Transthoracic echocardiography (transthoracic scan of the cardiac chambers). Sometimes called "echocardioscopy," to underline the concept of problem-tailored imaging instead of the complex diagnostic parameters evaluated by a US cardiac specialist, it may allow direct or indirect visualization of the tip. A

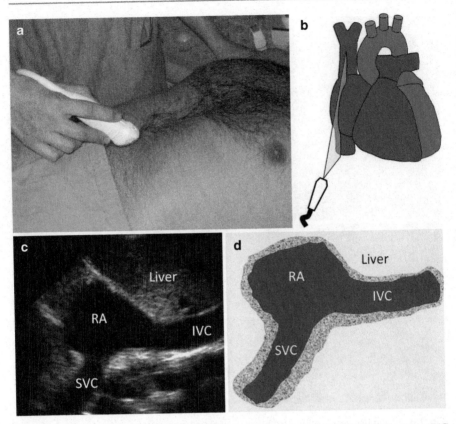

Fig. 7.4 Atrio-bicaval view obtained by subcostal ultrasound scan of the cardiac chambers: *IVC* inferior vena cava; *RA* right atrium; *SVC* superior vena cava. (**a**) Probe position on patient. (**b**) Schematic explanation of the subcostal scanning. (**c**) Ultrasound image. (**d**) Schematic interpretation of the ultrasound image

medium- or low-frequency probe is placed on the chest wall, either in the parasternal, apical, or subcostal approach, to visualize the right atrial chamber, possibly the terminal segments of the superior and inferior venae cavae and the catheter/guidewire within them (Fig. 7.4).

– Direct visualization: the tip is directly visualized within the cardiac chambers [25–27].
– Indirect visualization by contrast-enhanced ultrasound: 5 ml of a saline-air mixture, prepared with two 10-mL syringes containing one 9 mL of saline and the other 1 mL of air, is injected rapidly as a bolus through the catheter so that a stream of microbubbles can be seen through its tip, to assess positioning. Standardized parameters, such as appearance within 2 s of a flush of bubbles coming from the SVC, allow to estimate the distance of the tip from the atriocaval junction [28]. This technique is approved by international guidelines [29].

• Supraclavicular scan: this is an uncommon but promising scanning view performed with a microconvex intermediate medium-/high-frequency probe through a supraclavicular window. This approach combines the scanning depth of a convex

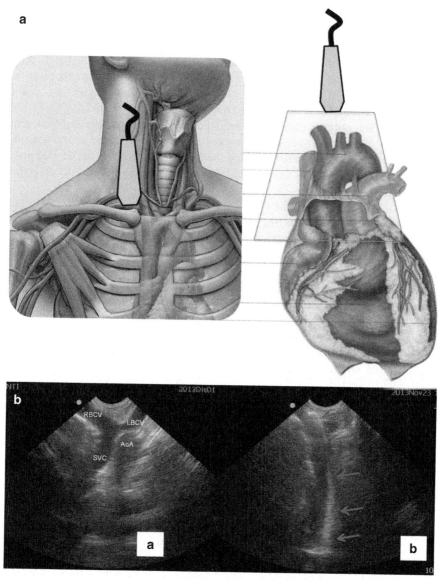

Fig. 7.5 Coronal ultrasound scan of brachiocephalic-caval venous axis via a supraclavicular window using a microconvex probe. (**a**) Schematic view (Courtesy of Teleflex - modified). (**b**) Ultrasound images: *a* – pre-procedural anatomy: *RBCV* right brachiocephalic vein, *LBCV* left brachiocephalic vein, *SVC* superior vena cava, *AoA* aortic arch. *b* – Intra-procedural view: catheter within the SVC (*arrows*) (Author's personal cases)

medium-frequency probe with the good resolution of a linear high-frequency one and the good maneuverability of a small-tipped probe in the narrow space of the supraclavicular fossa. This allows scanning the brachiocephalic-caval venous axis in a coronal fashion in order to visualize the entire catheter/guidewire within the great vessels and locate the tip within the lower SVC [30, 31] (Fig. 7.5).

Further interesting developments in this field are related to the application of real-time multidimensional ultrasound to vascular access [32, 33].

Advantages of ultrasound for tip location are the possibility of performing the diagnostic test during or after the insertion procedure and documenting the tip position as an image on a physical support. The main disadvantages are related to the low reproducibility of the diagnostic test due to eventual problems with the acoustic windows and the high level of expertise required.

Negative and positive assessment techniques, evaluating catheter direction plus tip location, can be combined to improve accuracy of ultrasound in preventing primary malposition and accurately placing the tip of the catheter in the desired position and may be part of a multiprocedural protocol for tip control (see later on in this chapter).

Even if it is not the case for PICC insertion, which does not carry a significant risk of pleural complications, the possibility to rule out pneumothorax or pleural collections after insertion of a central line is responsible for the increasing spread of ultrasound use in association with vascular access procedures [26, 28].

7.4.2.4 Transesophageal Echocardiography (TEE)

Transesophageal echocardiography allows a direct visualization of the tip within the atriocaval region and is the most accurate tool to evaluate its actual position. After obtaining the so-called atrio-bicaval view, the atriocaval junction is identified looking at the crista terminalis, a round-shaped fibromuscular labrum originating from the interatrial septum and running anteriorly to the atrial orifice of the SVC. It is seen as a hyperechoic spur abutting in the right atrium at the SVC inlet. This structure is the residual scar of the embryologic fusion between the caval sinus and the properly called right atrium, thus representing an unequivocal anatomical landmark of the SVC inlet into the right atrium. Tip relationships with the atriocaval junction may be precisely and quantitatively estimated in terms of centimeters from the crista terminalis [34–37]. Despite its very high accuracy, TEE is only feasible in anesthetized patients and is thus of little value in clinical practice, especially for PICC insertion procedures, usually performed bedside in awake patients.

7.4.2.5 Intracavitary Electrocardiography

The position of the tip inside the venous system can be detected by regarding the catheter itself (or a guidewire inside the catheter) as an intracavitary electrode which replaces the 'red' or "right shoulder" ' electrode (lead II in a bipolar three-lead EKG setting according to the classical Einthoven triangle) of the standard surface EKG. When the EKG monitor is connected to the intracavitary electrode, the reading of lead II will show a P wave whose shape and height will change while advancing the catheter within the venous system towards the heart.

This method was first described in 1949 [38]. After the first experiences in the 1960s, it was accepted in clinical practice in the 1980s and is now widely used in Europe (specifically in Germany and in Italy) for positioning the tip of different types of central venous access devices in adults [10]; in a few cases, the method has also been tested in neonates [39–42], for positioning the tip of umbilical catheters and epicutaneo-caval catheters, and even applied in difficult clinical situations, such as atrial fibrillation or other cardiac arrhythmias, where atrial electrical activity is uncoordinated and does not result in a single P wave [43, 44].

Intracavitary EKG uses the catheter itself as an intracavitary (endovascular) electrode. It allows locating the atriocaval junction and its surroundings by the shape and height modifications of the P wave that the intravascular electrode detects while it is advanced from the peripheral venous system towards the heart. The DII lead (right shoulder–left leg) should be used, since in this lead the variations of the P wave are particularly evident (the electrical axis of the right atrium is oriented similarly to the DII axis in the Einthoven's triangle). Amplitude variations of the P wave reflect the closeness of the intravascular electrode to the electrical field originated by the right atrium, and generally speaking, the more the intracavitary electrode is close to the right atrium, the more the P wave will appear high peaked. More specifically, while the intravascular electrode is advanced, the P wave:

- Increases in size while approaching the right atrium
- Reaches a maximum at the entrance in the RA
- Decreases and becomes biphasic when placed deep in the RA
- Becomes negative while leaving the atrium to enter the inferior vena cava
- Becomes similar to a surface-recorded ventricular ectopic beat if the right ventricle is entered instead of the inferior vena cava

Anatomical-electrophysiological correlation studies have demonstrated that the P wave amplitude and shape variation patterns, while advancing the intravascular electrode within the venous system towards the heart, are related to the tip position as follows [34–37, 45]:

- Intracavitary electrode outside the superior vena cava: the P wave is as high as the one recorded from the surface, that is, from the skin electrodes.
- SVC (superior one-third): the P wave starts increasing in amplitude.
- SVC (superior-medium one-third): P wave = 1/3 of the maximal P wave.
- SVC (medium-lower one-third): endocavitary P wave = 1/2 of the maximal P wave.
- SVC close (about 1 cm) to the RA: endocavitary $P = 2/3$ of the maximal P wave.
- Atriocaval junction (tip at the entrance of the right atrium) = first appearing maximal P wave.
- RA (superior one-third): endocavitary P = persistent maximal P wave (visible for 1–3 cm of the intravenous track).
- Deep atrium = P wave decreases and then becomes biphasic.
- IVC = negative endocavitary P wave.
- Right ventricle: "ventricular ectopic beat"-shaped P wave (Fig. 7.6).

If no variations in the P wave amplitude can be seen, we can assume that the tip of the catheter/endovascular electrode has not reached the atriocaval region and is thus malpositioned. Note that if not any modification of the P wave can be seen, the actual position of the catheter tip cannot be established, but the method still gives an essential information: likely, the tip is not in the right place.

A full description of the technical details of the method is not in the scope of this chapter and is available elsewhere.

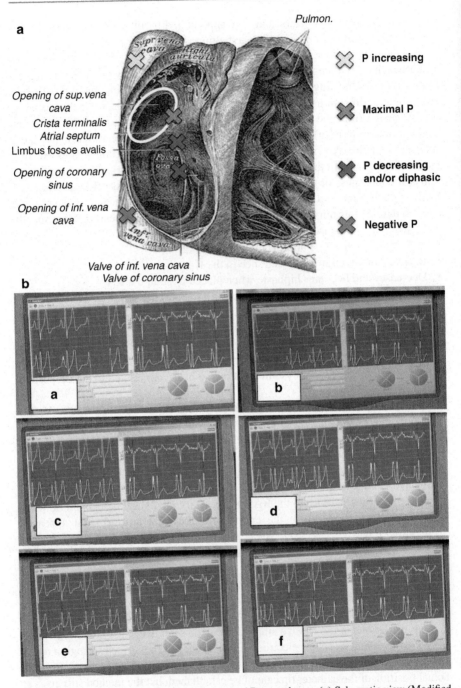

Fig. 7.6 Correlation between cardiac anatomy and P wave shapes. (**a**) Schematic view (Modified from [49]). (**b**) Endocavitary EKG (*yellow trace*, left part of the screen) as compared to the surface (*white trace*, left part of the screen). *a* – endocavitary p equal to the surface one. *b* – endocavitary P wave starting to increase while advancing the catheter/endocavitary electrode. *c* – maximal endocavitary P wave. *d* – endocavitary P wave=2/3 of the maximal. *e* – biphasic endocavitary P wave. *f* – negative endocavitary P wave. The right part of the screen is dedicated to frozen images (Author's personal cases). See text for details and anatomical correlations

Many papers from the last 20 years have proven the EKG method to be as accurate as the radiologic methods, considering that the "gold standard" of accuracy is possibly the TEE, which cannot be routinely adopted because of its invasiveness. A comprehensive review of literature has been provided in a previous paper from our working group [10]. In fact, the accuracy of intra-procedural fluoroscopy and of post-procedural chest X-ray is not 100 %, since many factors may alter the interpretation of the radiologic image (artifacts, errors of perspective, technical difficulties especially in bedridden patients, etc.), leading to a significant incidence of false-positive and false-negative diagnoses. On the other hand, a recent Italian multicenter study on adult patients has demonstrated that the intracavitary EKG method is safe and feasible in almost 100 % of those patients whose P wave is identifiable at the basal surface EKG, with an overall accuracy as high as 95 %, comparable with fluoroscopy [21]. Similar preliminary results have been documented in a recently closed Italian multicenter study on pediatric patients (submitted data).

Future evolution of the method regards improving easiness of use and widening the range of patients that may benefit from it. New dedicated devices have been introduced in clinical practice:

- "Guided" and/or "user-friendly" EKG-only based devices to improve interpretation of the EKG trace. Most of these devices, such as Sapiens TLS Tip locator System® (Bard Access Systems Inc.), Nautilus® (Vygon), and Celerity® (Medcomp), consist of a hardware enabling a standard laptop PC (or a different dedicated device) to detect the EKG trace plus a software allowing the operator to dialogue with the laptop manipulating the detected signals: freezing, saving, measuring, comparing different waves, printing (EKG traces and or detailed labels), and even more options may improve reading, interpretation, and documentation of the intracavitary EKG (Fig. 7.7). Some of these devices even allow complex calculations such as the area below the atrial signal, representing the total amount

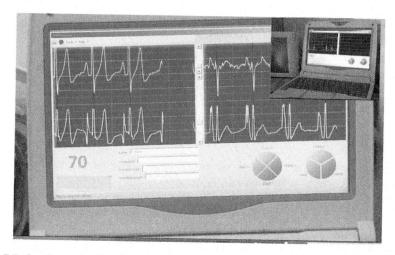

Fig. 7.7 Small computer-based EKG monitor: left part of the screen dedicated to the dynamic EKG monitoring; right side for freezing; yellow trace = endocavitary; white trace = surface

of atrial energy (instead of the simple amplitude of the P wave) detected by the electrode in its various positions within the vascular system, a parameter whose implication may be further developed in the next future to better standardize the EKG method in situation with impaired P waves as described ahead.

- EKG+navigation integrated devices to improve applicability and accuracy of the EKG method. These devices add to the EKG method that still gives the main parameter to locate the tip of the catheter, a "navigation" technology in the same machine.
  - Vasonova Vascular Positioning System (VPS)® (Teleflex). The added technology is Doppler based. The Doppler signal, released and perceived by a specific transducer mounted on the stylet within the catheter, alerts the operator when the catheter runs against the blood flow, thus meaning that a misdirection is ongoing; the system works with a multiparametric screen that includes the endocavitary EKG trace, the original Doppler signal, and a simple "traffic light-like" dynamic icon helping the operator to interpret Doppler (catheter direction) and EKG (final tip position).
  - CatFinder® (Elcam). The added technology is presso-acoustic based. A transducer applied on the catheter hub perceives the pressure wave coming from the cardiac chambers during their mechanical activity. The pressure wave is assumed to start synchronously with the cardiac electrical activity, and the time delay to reach the transducer is used to calculate the distance of the tip from the origin of the pressure wave (i.e., the cardiac chamber).
  - Sherlock 3CG® (Bard Access Systems Inc.). The added technology is electromagnetic based, such as in the devices previously described. The operator can follow the direction of the catheter (i.e., the magnetic stylet within it) as detected by the sensor placed on the chest wall and represented in a multiparametric screen that includes the intracavitary EKG trace as well (Fig. 7.8).

The EKG method has several advantages:

- Safety for the patient.
- Applicability to all kinds of catheters (even to separately control different lumens of a multi-lumen catheter).
- High accuracy.
- Quickness (as opposed to the time-consuming control by intra-procedural fluoroscopy) and easiness (if compared to training in the use and interpretation of radiologic imaging).
- "Real-time" verification of the position of the tip, avoiding resorting to postprocedural repositioning maneuvers (complicated, expensive, and potentially risky).
- Applicability of the method days, weeks, or months after insertion in order to verify the correct tip position.
- Documentability of the tip location by printing out the intracavitary EKG reading or using specific labeling softwares included in the above-described dedicated devices.
- Applicability in clinical situations where radiologic verification is contraindicated (pregnancy) or logistically difficult (PICC insertion at home or in a hospice).

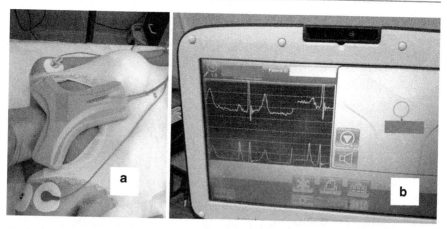

Fig. 7.8 Electromagnetic tracking + endocavitary EKG: note the sensor applied on the chest wall (**a**) and the separated mutiparametric screen showing both endocavitary EKG and the tracking results (**b**)

- Inexpensiveness: it can be performed with minimal costs (cable, wires, transducer, and the availability of an EKG monitor), especially if compared to intra-procedural fluoroscopy.
- Convenience: intra-procedural verification of the position of the tip avoids expensive and time-consuming maneuvers related to the repositioning of a catheter whose malposition has been diagnosed on a post-procedural chest X-ray.

The most important limits of the EKG method remain related to a few amount of patients (7 %) bearing an aberrant or no identifiable P wave at the basal surface EKG (predominantly atrial fibrillation, but even junctional rhythms or other complex electrical atrial dysfunctions) or an indwelling and functioning pacemaker [21]. Recent researches in this field are aimed at finding parameters that allow application of the method to dysrhythmic patients. As a matter of fact, an endocavitary atrial activity with clear differences from the surface EKG is still identifiable in most patients with atrial dysrhythmias (Fig. 7.9) when the catheter enters the right atrium [43, 44]. In a pilot study carried out in our center, the EKG method – as performed with a digital EKG-based system, which offers not only the wave form pattern but also the total amount of electrical energy recorded by the electrode – was effective in locating the catheter tip at the cavo-atrial junction in 15/16 atrial fibrillation patients. Thus, endocavitary EKG may still be used at least to confirm that the catheter has grossly reached the atriocaval region. Introduction of digital systems (see above) may further improve in the next future the results of the method in AF patients after identification of quantifiable, standardizable, and universally applicable EKG-based parameters, such as energy (the area below the atrial trace at EKG) instead of simple P wave amplitude [44].

As concerns patients with active pacemakers, the intracavitary EKG method is normally applicable if the pacing device is not working during the insertion procedure (on demand devices), while, if working, its signal covers every spontaneous

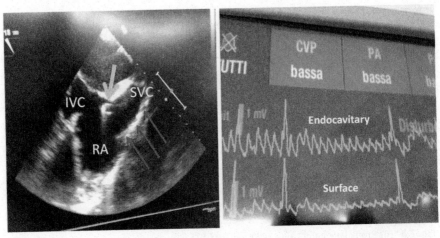

Fig. 7.9 Comparison between endocavitary EKG and transesophageal echocardiography in a patient with atrial fibrillation. (**a**) Transesophageal echocardiography: J-tipped guidewire at the atriocaval junction (*yellow arrow*), crista terminalis (*red arrows*), *IVC* inferior vena cava, *RA* right atrium, *SVC* superior vena cava. (**b**) Correspondent EKG: see the high-voltage activity in the endocavitary trace

atrial activity and does not allow to detect any variations while approaching the cardiac chambers with the catheter. For this small amount of patients, an additional tip location method should be used, and a protocol that still allows avoiding X-ray-based procedures can be proposed as shown later on.

7.5 Documentation Issues

The final position of the tip should be documented, both for patient's safety and for medical legal protection of the operator. In some countries, such as in Italy, a written description of the procedure is enough for medical legal purposes, but this may not happen in other countries. Moreover, from a clinical point of view, documentation has a critical role in allowing an operator who was not involved in the insertion procedure to directly evaluate the primary post-procedural tip position and, ideally, to repeat the diagnostic procedure comparing the results with the peri-implantation ones. From both clinical and legal point of view, this is of paramount importance if a suspicion of secondary malposition occurs, especially if the patient is assisted in a different center from the one involved in the implantation procedure.

In this respect, endocavitary EKG is, at present, the only alternative to fluoroscopy (if we exclude transesophageal echocardiography which is inapplicable in awake patients) in giving the chance of documenting the procedure and the final tip position, with multiple options:

- Describing the height of the P wave quantified in millimeters (at present not suitable for patients with atrial fibrillation, as long as other quantifiable parameters, such as energy, are not standardized yet with respect of their accuracy and reproducibility in determining the relationship of the tip with the atriocaval region)

- Including a paper-based intracavitary EKG trace in the patient record
- Including a digital recording of the EKG trace in the patient record, on a physical support or online, where this facility is available

The last two options are feasible even for patients with atrial fibrillation. If another intra-procedural method is adopted, one should be aware that most of them are unable to locate the tip in respect to its anatomical surroundings, so that a post-procedural X-ray is still needed.

7.6 The Future of Tip Verification

As long as X-ray-based verification is recommended as the gold standard [6], different methods should be approved at least as a local policy, ideally in a wide national or international consensus [46]. In this respect, endocavitary EKG is a good alternative to radiologic verification of tip position, as recently recognized by medical societies [47] and international guidelines [5].

If endocavitary EKG is used, a post-procedural chest X-ray can be completely avoided provided that [5]:

- Tip location was clearly determined according to the approved protocol.
- A pleural complication can be excluded anyway; this may appear obvious for PICC insertion, a procedure virtually free from this kind of complications, but is of critical importance while placing central lines with a cervicothoracic approach; in this respect, transthoracic ultrasound may help excluding PNX and/or pleural fluid collections, with a very high accuracy in trained hands [28, 48].

As part of a multiprocedural protocol for verifying tip position, endocavitary EKG may substantially decrease, and ultimately abolish, the need for X-ray-based controls [49].

Our present protocol for confirming tip position is shown in Fig. 7.10.

In order to avoid radiologic confirmation of tip position in all patients, an advanced multiprocedural protocol may be proposed and validated in the next future, as shown in Fig. 7.11.

Conclusions

Tip position is of paramount importance and should be verified before starting infusion on any central venous line.

Intra-procedural methods for verifying the location of the tip are to be preferred, since they avoid the risks, delays, and costs of repositioning the tip.

Among the intra-procedural methods, fluoroscopy is still the gold standard, though cost-related and logistic issues may limit its use in high-volume centers and in a high proportion of patients who undergo the insertion procedure bedside or in outpatient settings.

Alternative intra-procedural methods include intracavitary EKG and electromagnetic-based and ultrasound-based tip location techniques. The intracavitary EKG appears to be the safest, cheapest, most accurate, and universally applicable method. Its limits may be overcome by adopting an integrated

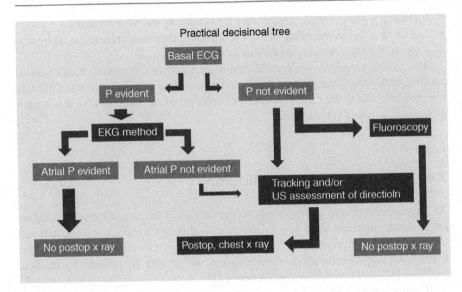

Fig. 7.10 Decisional algorithm used by the author's working group

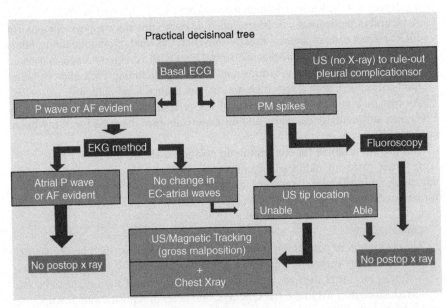

Fig. 7.11 Proposal of advanced multiprocedural protocol (to be validated) for tip position control

multiprocedural protocol including "predictive" methods as well as ultrasound and/or electromagnetic tracking-based tip location techniques in order to completely avoid X-ray-based procedures according to the most recent recommendations for patient's safety [24].

References

1. Cl N (2007) Reduction of malposition in peripherally inserted central catheters with tip location system. JAVA 12:29–31
2. Vesely TM (2003) Central venous catheter tip position: a continuing controversy. J Vasc Interv Radiol 14:527–534
3. NAVAN – National Association of Vascular Access Networks (1998) NAVAN position statement on terminal tip placement. J Vasc Access Dev 3:8–10
4. Bishop L, Dougherty L, Bodenham A, Mansi J, Crowes P, Kibbler C, Shannon M, Treleave J, BCSH Committee (2007) Guidelines on the insertion and management of central venous access devices in adults. Int J Lab Hem 29:261–278
5. Pittiruti M, Hamilton H, Biffi R, MacFie J, Pertkiewiz M (2009) ESPEN guidelines on parenteral nutrition: central venous catheters (access, care, diagnosis and therapy of complications). Clin Nutr 28:365–377
6. Infusion Nurses Society (2011) Infusion nursing standards of practice. J Infus Nurs 34 (1 Suppl):S1–S110
7. Petersen J, Delaney JH, Brakstad MT, Rowbotham RK, Bagley CM Jr (1999) Silicone venous access devices positioned with their tips high in the superior vena cava are more likely to malfunction. Am J Surg 178:38–41
8. Caers J, Fontaine C, Vinh-Hung V et al (2005) Catheter tip position as a risk factor for thrombosis associated with the use of subcutaneous infusion ports. Support Care Cancer 13: 325–331
9. McGee DC, Gould MK (2003) Preventing complications of central venous catheterization. N Engl J Med 348:1123–1133
10. Pittiruti M, La Greca A, Scoppettuolo G (2011) The electrocardiographic method for positioning the tip of central venous catheters. J Vasc Access 12(4):280–291
11. Puel V, Caudry M, le Métayer P et al (1993) Superior vena cava thrombosis related to catheter malposition in cancer chemotherapy given through implanted ports. Cancer 72:2248–2252
12. Taylor RW, Palagiri AV (2007) Central venous catheterization. Crit Care Med 35:1390–1396
13. Peres PW (1990) Positioning central venous catheters - a prospective survey. Anaesth Intensive Care 18:536–539
14. Kim H, Jeong CH, Byon HJ, Shin HK, Yun TJ, Lee JH, Park YH, Kim JT (2013) Predicting the optimal depth of left-sided central venous catheters in children. Anaesthesia 68(10): 1033–1037
15. Yoon SZ, Shin TJ, Kim HS, Lee J, Kim CS, Kim SD, Park CD (2006) Depth of a central venous catheter tip: length of insertion guideline for pediatric patients. Acta Anaesthesiol Scand 50(3):355–357
16. Kim JH, Kim CS, Bahk JH, Cha KJ, Park YS, Jeon YT, Han SH (2005) The optimal depth of central venous catheter for infants less than 5 kg. Anesth Analg 101(5):1301–1303
17. Andropoulos DB, Bent ST, Skjonsby B, Stayer SA (2001) The optimal length of insertion of central venous catheters for pediatric patients. Anesth Analg 93(4):883–886
18. Lum P (2004) A New formula-based measurement guide for optimal positioning of central venous catheters. JAVA 9(2):80–85
19. Schweickert WD, Herlitz J, Pohlman AS, Gehlbach BK, Hall JB, Kress JP (2009) A randomized, controlled trial evaluating postinsertion neck ultrasound in peripherally inserted central catheter procedures. Crit Care Med 37(4):1217–1221
20. Royer T, Earhart A (2007) Taking the leap from PICC placement to tip placement. JAVA 12:148–155
21. Pittiruti M, Bertollo D, Briglia E, Buononato M, Capozzoli G, De Simone L, La Greca A, Pelagatti C, Sette P (2012) The intracavitary EKG method for positioning the tip of central venous catheters: results of an Italian multicenter study. J Vasc Access 13(3):357–365
22. Aslamy Z, Cl D, Heffner JE (1998) MRI of central venous anatomy: implications for central venous catheter insertion. Chest 114:820–826

23. Claasz AA, Chorley DP (2007) A study of the relationship of the superior vena cava to the bony landmarks of the sternum in the supine adult: implications for magnetic guidance systems. JAVA 12(3):132–139

24. Shekelle PG, Pronovost PJ, Wachter RM et al (2013) The top patient safety strategies that can be encouraged for adoption now. Ann Intern Med 158(5 Pt 2):365–368

25. Maury E, Guglielminotti J, Alzieu M, Guidet B, Offenstadt G (2001) Ultrasonic examination: an alternative to chest radiography after central venous catheter insertion? Am J Respir Crit Care Med 164(3):403–5

26. Bedel J, Vallée F, Mari A, Riu B, Planquette B, Geeraerts T, Génestal M, Minville V, Fourcade O (2013) Guidewire localization by transthoracic echocardiography during central venous catheter insertion: a periprocedural method to evaluate catheter placement. Intensive Care Med 39(11):1932–1937

27. Vezzani A, Brusasco C, Palermo S, Launo C, Mergoni M, Corradi F (2010) Ultrasound localization of central vein catheter and detection of postprocedural pneumothorax: an alternative to chest radiography. Crit Care Med 38(2):533–538

28. Lamperti M, Bodenham AR, Pittiruti M, Blaivas M, Augoustides JG, Elbarbary M, Pirotte T, Karakitsos D, Ledonne J, Doniger S, Scoppettuolo G, Feller-Kopman D, Schummer W, Biffi R, Desruennes E, Melniker LA, Verghese ST (2012) International evidence-based recommendations on ultrasound-guided vascular access. Intensive Care Med 38(7):1105–1117

29. La Greca A (2013) Current recommendations for placement of long term VADs: role of ultrasound, role of intracavitary EKG and the SILTA-2 bundle in 2013. Proceedings 8th GAVeCeLT congress, Turin, 6–7th Dec 2013 (in press)

30. Biasucci DG (2013) Ultrasound for tip verification and for early detection of pleural complications. Proceedings 8th GAVeCeLT congress, Turin, 6–7th Dec 2013 (in press)

31. French JL, Raine-Fenning NJ, Hardman JG, Bedforth NM (2008) Pitfalls of ultrasound guided vascular access: the use of three/four-dimensional ultrasound. Anaesthesia 63(8):806–813

32. Dowling M, Jlala HA, Hardman JG, Bedforth NM (2011) Real-time three-dimensional ultrasound-guided central venous catheter placement. Anesth Analg 112(2):378–381

33. Chu KS, Hsu JH, Wang SS et al (2004) Accurate central venous port-A catheter placement: intravenous electrocardiography and surface landmark techniques compared by using transesophageal echocardiography. Anesth Analg 98:910–914

34. Hsu JH, Wang CK, Chu KS et al (2006) Comparison of radiographic landmarks and the echocardiographic SVC/RA junction in the positioning of long term central venous catheters. Acta Anaesthesiol Scand 50:731–735

35. Jeon Y, Ryu HG, Yoon SZ, Kim JH, Bahk JH (2006) Transesophageal echocardiographic evaluation of EKG-guided central venous catheter placement. Can J Anaesth 53(10):978–983

36. Yunseok J, Ho-Geol R, Seun-Zhoo Y, Jim-Hee K, Jae-Hyon B (2006) Transesophageal echocardiographic evaluation of EKG- guided central venous catheter placement. Can J Anaesth 53:978–983

37. Hellerstein HK, Pritchard WH, Lewis RL (1949) Recording of intracavitary potentials through a single-lumen saline filled cardiac catheter. Proc Soc Exp Biol Med 71:58–60

38. Neubauer AP (1995) Percutaneous central IV access in the neonate: experience with 535 silastic catheters. Acta Pediatr 84:758–760

39. Lozano LS, Capdevila MB (1997) Cateters de silastic: localizacion del extremo distal mediante monitorizacion electrocardiografica. Rev Enferm 20(230):50–52

40. Biban P, Cavalli C, Santuz P, Soffiati M, Rugolotto S, Zangardi T (2000) Positioning of umbilical vein catheter with EKG-guided technique: randomized study. Acta Biomed Ateneo Parmense 71(suppl):647–650

41. Tierney SN, Katke J, Langer JC (2000) Cost comparison of electro- cardiography versus fluoroscopy for central venous line positioning in children. J Am Coll Surg 191:209–211

42. Engelhardt W, Sold M, Helzel MV (1989) EKG-controlled placement of central venous catheters in patients with atrial fibrillation. Anaesthesist 38:476–479

43. Pittiruti M, La Greca A, Scoppettuolo G, et al. (2011) EKG-controlled placement of central venous catheters in patients with atrial fibrillation. Proceedings of the INS 2011 annual convention & industrial exhibition, Louisville, 21–26 May 2011
44. Ender J, Erdoes G, Krohmer E, Olthoff D, Mukherjee C (2009) Transesophageal echocardiography for verification of the position of the electrocardiographically-placed central. J Cardiothorac Vasc Anesth 23(4):457–461
45. Gebhard RE (2007) Can electrocardiogram-controlled central line placement decrease the need for routine chest radiographs after central venous cannulation? Anesth Analg 104:1614
46. Weissauer W (1998) Der Cava-Katheter aus medico-legaler Sicht. Anaesthesiol Intensivmed Notfallmed Schmerzther 33:117
47. Volpicelli G, Elbarbary M, Blaivas M et al (2012) International evidence-based recommendations for point-of-care lung ultrasound. Intensive Care Med 38(4):577–591
48. Antonaglia V, Ristagno G, Berlot G (2008) Procedural and clinical data plus electrocardiographic guidance greatly reduce the need for routine chest radiograph following central line placement. J Trauma 64(4):1146
49. Gray H (1918) Anatomy of the human body. Lea & Febiger, Philadelphia

Frequency, Diagnosis, and Management of Occlusive and Mechanical PICC Complications

8

Lisa Dougherty

8.1 Catheter Occlusions

Patency is defined as the ability to infuse through and aspirate blood from a VAD [1]. It is important at all times for the patency of the PICC to be maintained. *Occlusion* predisposes the PICC to device damage, infection, disruption to medication delivery, and inconvenience to patients.

PICCs may become occluded because of the following:
1. Thrombotic: (a) Blood clot within the lumen or (b) fibrin sheath/tail
2. Non-thrombotic: (a) Precipitation of drugs or (b) mechanical causes [1]

8.2 Types

There are two main types of occlusion:
1. Partial (*persistent withdrawal occlusion*) is when the catheter will flush but will not enable the practitioner to withdraw blood, which may affect the ability to gain a sample and more importantly may prevent the practitioner from checking patency of the device [2].
2. Complete (*total occlusion*) is when there is an inability to withdraw blood and infuse or inject into the catheter [3, 4].

8.3 Incidence

Occlusions occur in 14–36 % of patients within 1–2 years of catheter placement and may occur in 50 % of children and 66 % of adults with a long-term CVC [3, 4]. Before effective interventions, 25 % of all catheters placed were removed due to

L. Dougherty
The Royal Marsden NHS Foundation Trust, Downs Road, Sutton, Surrey Su2 5PT, UK
e-mail: lisa.dougherty@rmh.nhs.uk

S. Sandrucci, B. Mussa (eds.), *Peripherally Inserted Central Venous Catheters*,
DOI 10.1007/978-88-470-5665-7_8, © Springer-Verlag Italia 2014

catheter-related occlusions – of these 58 % were thrombotic and 42 % non-thrombotic/ mechanical [1]. The incidence of thrombosis can be between 1 and 5 % [5], with rates in PICCs 4–5 % [6, 7] . There is an increased risk in suboptimal tip position, with the risk decreasing using small-bore catheters, the use of the basilic rather than cephalic vein, and those who have had a past history of venous thromboembolism [8].

8.4   Diagnosis

The first step to management is to ascertain the cause of occlusion:
- Assess catheter function – flow of infusion/ability to aspirate blood.
- External occlusion – kinking/clamps, etc.
- Postural changes – relieved when position changed.
- Relevant catheter use – history of what was infused, blood products.
- Physical assessment – assess patients for signs of edema, redness, pain, or dilated vessels.
  Baskin et al. suggest that the practitioner should rule out mechanical, then precipitate, and then thrombotic causes [3].

8.5   Non-thrombotic Occlusions

These account for 5 % of all catheter occlusions [9]. Causes can be:

8.5.1   Mechanical

- External clamps inadvertently left closed
- Kinking of catheter tubing
- Constricting sutures
- Catheter tip blocked by a blood vessel wall
- Dislodged or malpositioned port needles
- *Pinch-off syndrome* (which causes it in 1.1 % of patients but unlikely with PICCs) [4]
  External clamps should be checked to ensure they are open and that the catheter is not kinked under dressing or within securement device; remove any constricting sutures (and resuture to skin if necessary) or change to an adhesive securing device and ask the patient to change their position such as deep breathing, lifting arm [10].

8.5.2   Precipitation

Precipitates can form within the catheter lumen following administration of minerals, lipids, or chemically incompatible medications [4]. Mixing of incompatible medications may occur when medications are not flushed adequately. Solubility is highly dependent on drug concentration and pH. IV lipid, calcium salts, and phosphate complexes as well as antibiotics can all result in precipitate formation. Lipid occlusion may slowly accumulate within the catheter lumen presenting as resistance to flushing over several days before complete occlusion [10].

There are a number of agents, which can be used to help dissolve drug or lipid precipitation. *Sodium bicarbonate* can be used for medication that precipitates in an acidic environment [4]. For mineral occlusions, for example, lipids in parenteral nutrition, *hydrochloric acid* can be used effectively [4]. *Ethanol* has also been used with catheters occluded with fat emulsion, but there are concerns about all alcohol solutions in catheters made polyurethane. Prior to use, the manufacturer should be contacted for guidance in their safe use and compatibility with the vascular access device

8.6   Thrombotic Occlusions

The main types of thrombotic occlusions

8.6.1   Intraluminal Thrombus

These occur as partial occlusions and account for 5–25 % of all catheter occlusion [3, 11]. They can result from:
(a) Inadequate or poor technique when flushing (i.e., not using positive pressure)
(b) Inadequate flow through lumens of the catheter; allowing an infusion to run dry – which allows blood to track back up the tubing or switching off of an infusion without flushing
(c) Reflux from changes in intrathoracic pressure, coughing, congestive heart failure, heavy lifting, and frequent withdrawal of blood via catheter [20]
These may cause sluggish flow apparent on flushing or infusing solutions [12].

8.6.2   Fibrin Tail/Sheath

This is extraluminal occurring when fibrin adheres to the external surface of the catheter within 24 h following CVC placement and usually develops within 2 weeks [3]. The fibrin, blood cell, and platelet adhere to the end of the catheter and form a tail or sheath. The tail becomes longer as more cells and other blood products are progressively deposited. A fibrin sleeve may resemble a sock and encase the whole catheter at the tip, and this may extend along the entire catheter to the point where the catheter exits onto the skin. It acts as a one-way valve and allows the catheter to flush but does not allow blood to be aspirated [11].

The consequences of fibrins sheaths are as follows:
1. Elimination of catheter function
2. Can be seeded with bacteria and microorganisms which can then be disseminated into the bloodstream when the catheter is flushed or aspirated
3. Extravasation – medication or fluid backtracks along the outside portion and exits out of venous entry site and into the surrounding tissues [2, 13]

8.6.3 Mural Thrombus

These may form when the catheter tip causes vessel wall injury, and fibrin from the vessel wall injury attracts to the fibrin building on the catheter surface. While it is not significant in itself, it can increase the potential risk of venous thrombosis. A *venous thrombosis* is a clot of blood that can be present at the tip of a catheter or can surround the catheter, for example, a thrombosis in the upper arm caused by the presence of a PICC.

8.6.4 Frequency

The incidence of thrombotic catheter dysfunction is between 3 and 7 %. It depends on the type of illness, type of catheter, and duration of catheter in situ. The risk is increased if the tip is high in the SVC and brachiocephalic vein (incidence 75 %) [8, 9].

8.6.5 Prevention

Two main types of solutions are used to maintain patency in VADs: *heparin* and 0.9 % sodium chloride. All devices should be flushed with 10–20 mL *0.9 % sodium chloride* after blood withdrawal followed by the appropriate flushing solution [1, 14, 15].

Maintaining patency can be achieved by:

- A continuous infusion to keep the vein open (*KVO*), either by the patient being attached to an infusion of 0.9 % sodium chloride via a volumetric pump, which reduces comfort and mobility, or by use of an elastomeric device, which is less restrictive and has been able to reduce loss of patency by 50 % [16]
- Intermittent flushing (previously known as a "heparin lock")

When used for intermittent therapy, the device should be flushed after each use with the appropriate flushing solution [1]. There is still no consensus about the solution to use or frequency of flushing [17, 18] as the evidence is not adequate to make definitive conclusions [19].

Heparinized saline is still a commonly accepted solution for maintaining the patency of CVCs for intermittent use or infrequent use [15]. The use of 0.9 % sodium chloride alone is becoming more common especially with valved catheters [14]. Using a 0.9 % sodium chloride flush avoids a number of issues with heparin such as cultural concerns, impact on coagulation laboratory values, drug incompatibility, bleeding, heparin-induced thrombocytopenia, and medication errors, so its use must be considered carefully [20, 21].

Flushing regimens, ranging from once daily to once weekly, have been found to be effective. However, using the correct techniques to flush the VAD has been highlighted as one of the key issues in maintaining patency [22, 23]. There are two stages in flushing:

1. Using a pulsated (push–pause) flush to create turbulent flow when administering the solution, regardless of type and volume. This removes debris from the internal catheter wall [23, 24].
2. The procedure is completed using the *positive-pressure technique*. This is accomplished by maintaining pressure on the plunger of the syringe while disconnecting the syringe from the injection cap, which prevents reflux of blood into the tip, reducing the risk of occlusion [14, 25].

Manufacturers have now produced *needleless injection caps* which aim to reduce occlusions and infection [26, 27, 28, 29]. A positive "displacement" cap can achieve positive pressure without practitioners being required to actively achieve the positive pressure [30]. They have been shown to significantly reduce the incidence of catheter occlusions [2, 31–33]. *Negative-pressure* devices require positive pressure on the syringe. *Neutral displacement* connectors are not dependent upon flushing technique and can be clamped before or after syringe disconnection [27].

Taurolidine inhibits and kills a wide range of organisms and can be used by instilling it into the catheter to prevent infection as they kill bacteria and prevent biofilm formation, which can occlude the catheter [34, 35]. *Heparin-bonded catheters* may reduce the risk of catheter-related thrombosis as well as catheter-related infections [36].

The use of *prophylactic anticoagulants* such as low-dose warfarin has been shown to be of no apparent benefit [37, 38]. However, if the patient has had previous thromboembolic events, full anticoagulation may be necessary [39].

8.6.6 Management

If the occlusion is caused by a clot, gentle pressure and aspiration may be sufficient to dislodge it. This should only be attempted using a 10 mL or larger syringe. *Smaller syringes* should never be used as they create a greater pressure [40, 41]. In order to enable the thrombolytic to be instilled without creating unnecessary pressure, a technique is used where a 3-way tap is attached so that a vacuum is created along one section, and then when the tap is turned towards the solution, it is "sucked" in without any undue pressure [42, 43]. Another method is use of the *percussion technique* [44].

8.6.6.1 Thrombotic Occlusions
In the case of a blood clot or fibrin causing the occlusion, the solution of choice is a thrombolytic agent. Anticoagulants, for example, heparin, are ineffective in restoring patency, but *low molecular weight heparin* can be used to manage thrombosis [8, 41].

Urokinase works by breaking down fibrin and thereby dissolving the clot. It was removed from the US market in 1998 due to potential risks of transmitting infectious agents, but it is still used in Europe. The usual dose is 10,000 units in 2 ml of sterle saline instilled into the catheter lumen every 10 minutes over a 30 minute period. Anecdotally practitioners have found it more effective if left for longer periods of time even over 24 h, although the potency of the drug decreases over time [10]. Recombinant urokinase has also been used successfully [19].

Alteplase has been used successfully in restoring patency to occluded catheter. Ponec et al. found that alteplase 2 mg per 2 ml was effective at restoring flow in catheters [45]. After 2 h of treatment, function was restored to 74 % of devices instilled with alteplase and only 17 % with placebo. After a 1–2-h treatment, 90 % function was resolved, and no serious drug-related adverse events were documented, concluding it was safe and effective. This was also supported by work carried out by Dietcher et al. and Timoney [46, 47].

Reteplase has been shown to clear 67–74 % of occlusions within 30–40 min and in 95 % of catheters overall [19]. Other newer agents include tenecteplase and alfimeprase, which may act more effectively and rapidly than current therapies in use, but Baskin et al. concluded that more randomized studies are required to determine optimal management of occluded catheters [19]. This is supported by the Cochrane review of interventions for restoring patency of occluded central venous catheter lumens. They found low- to very low-quality evidence suggesting that thrombolytic agents (urokinase and alteplase) could be effective in unblocking central venous catheters but concluded that more research is required to establish the efficacy and safety of different treatment interventions particularly in children [48].

8.7 Mechanical Complications

8.7.1 Catheter Damage

There are a number of causes of catheter fracture and subsequent embolism:
1. Forceful flushing in the presence of distal obstruction, manufacturing defect, or incorrect locking procedure
2. *Catheter shear* from needles/sutures or surgical instruments during insertion
3. On removal, using traction or against excessive resistance
4. Catheter pinch-off syndrome [49].
   Where the catheter damage occurs will dictate whether the catheter can be repaired or needs to be removed [10].
   Causes of *catheter damage* include:
(a) The catheter hub
   "Overscrewing" of a cap onto the hub and applying the cap to the hub which has been cleaned with alcohol but not allowed to dry adequately (which effectively "glues it on" causing difficulty when removing) can both result in cracking of the hub.
(b) Damage near the hub or below the bifurcation
   This can occur if the wrong types of *clamps* are used. Silicone is a fragile material and prone to damage; therefore, only the clamps provided with the catheter or smooth-bladed forceps should be used. Artery or toothed forceps can cause small breaks in the wall of the catheter [10].

(c) Damage higher up the catheter or above the bifurcation

This can occur on insertion and only be discovered once an infusion is commenced, but it more commonly occurs as a result of "nicking" the catheter when sutures are removed at the exit site or if small syringes are used to unblock a catheter, and the pressure results in small holes or splits in the catheter [10].

(d) Internal *catheter fracture*

This can result from damage caused during insertion by the practitioner but more commonly as a result of pinch-off syndrome [50, 51].

8.7.2   Prevention

Excessive force should never be used when flushing devices. When a catheter lumen is totally patent, internal pressure will not increase during flushing [49]. However, if resistance is felt (due to partial occlusion) and a force is applied to the plunger, particularly with a small-volume syringe, high pressure could result within the catheter, which may then rupture [41, 52, 53]. It is, therefore, recommended that the device is checked first with a 10 mL or larger syringe containing 0.9 % sodium chloride [15, 28, 52].

Damaged catheters result in removal of a working device, distress and discomfort for the patient, and time delay in treatment as well as cost. Prevention is the key and the use of the correct equipment when manipulating the catheter; managing occluded catheters appropriately and taking care when handling the catheter all help to prevent damage [50, 51].

- Check patency using 10 ml or larger syringes and avoid using smaller syringes wherever possible.
- Administer medication without force.
- Use correct types of clamps.
- Avoid using scissors or sharp objects around the catheter.
- Monitor catheters for pinholes, cuts, leaks, or tears.
- Check dressing for moisture or leaking at the insertion site during infusion and/ or injection.
- Educate the patient for the signs and symptoms to look out for and when to report [10].

8.7.3   Management

Immediate management would be to clamp the catheter and assess the degree of damage. Damaged catheters must be *repaired or removed* as any opening in the catheter can act as a potential entry for bacteria or air. The catheter can be shortened by cutting off the damaged portion and reapplying a new hub. This type of repair will need to be considered in respect to the tip location as shortening the catheter will result in a new tip location, and a chest x-ray must be performed to verify exact tip location [10, 50].

The ability to repair the hub will depend of the type of catheter as some have hubs which are integral to the catheter and cannot be repaired [10]. Any PICCs that can be repaired should be carried out in accordance with manufacturer's instructions [54]. Most PICCs have no repair segments commercially available, and so the best remedy is to exchange the catheter *over a guidewire*. This is performed by cutting the end off the catheter, threading a guidewire along the catheter to a specified distance, removal of the catheter, and the threading along of a new catheter. This can only be performed if there are no signs of infection [10].

If the catheter has *fractured*, a tourniquet under the arm during removal can "trap" the fragment in the periphery [55]. Removal of the catheter and retrieval of the fragment can be successfully carried out in interventional radiology. In the case of a PICC fracture, in order to retrieve the fragment, it may be necessary to perform a venous cutdown. If the fragment has migrated, then percutaneous removal or a thoracotomy may be necessary [50].

References

1. Dougherty L (2006) Central venous access devices. Blackwell Publishing, Oxford
2. Mayo DJ (2000) Catheter-related thrombosis. J Vasc Access Devices 5(2):10–20
3. Baskin JL et al (2011) Management of occlusion and thrombosis associated with long term indwelling central venous catheters. Lancet 374(9684):159
4. Doellman D (2011) Prevention, assessment and treatment of central venous occlusions in neonatal and young pediatric patients. J Infus Nurs 34(4):251–259
5. Qinming Z (2012) Chapter 23: Thrombosis. In: Di Carlo I, Biffi R (eds) Totally implantable venous access devices. Springer, Milan, pp 173–182
6. Lobo BL, Valdean G, Broyles J et al (2009) Risk of venous thromboembolism in hospitalized patients with peripherally inserted central catheters. J Hosp Med 4(7):417–422
7. Aw, A et al (2012) Incidence and predictive factors of symptomatic thrombosis related to peripherally inserted central catheters in chemotherapy patients. Thrombosis research 130(3): 323–326
8. Bodenham A, Simcock L (2009) Complications of central venous access. In: Hamilton H, Bodenham AR (eds) Central venous catheters. Wiley-Blackwell, Oxford, pp 175–205
9. Moureau N, Thompson McKinnon B, Douglas CM (1999) Multi disciplinary management of thrombotic catheter occlusions in vascular access devices. J Vasc Access Devices 4(2):22–29
10. Dougherty L, Watson J (2011) Vascular access devices. In: Dougherty L, Lister S (eds) The Royal Marsden Hospital manual of clinical nursing procedures, 8th edn. Wiley Publishing, Oxford
11. Kryswda ED (1999) Predisposing factors, prevention and management of central venous catheter occlusions. J Intraven Nurs 22(Suppl):S11–S17
12. Haire WD, Herbst SF (2000) Consensus statement on the use of t-PA to restore immediate function in the treatment of thrombotic catheter dysfunction. J Vasc Access Devices 5(2):28–36
13. Mayo DJ (1995) Chemotherapy extravasation: a consequence of fibrin sheath formation around venous access devices. Oncol Nurs Forum 22:(4)675–680
14. INS (2011) Infusion Nursing Standards of Practice 2011. J Infus Nurs 34(1):Suppl S1–S109
15. RCN (2010) Standards for infusion therapy, 3rd edn. Royal College of Nursing, London
16. Heath J, Jones S (2001) Utilization of an elastomeric continuous infusion device to maintain catheter patency. J Intraven Nurs 24(2):102–106

17. Mitchell MD, Anderson BJ, Williams K, Umscheid CA (2009) Heparin flushing and other interventions to maintain patency of central venous catheters: a systematic review. J Adv Nurs 65(10):2007–2021
18. Sona C, Prentice D, Schallom L (2011) National survey of CVC flushing in the intensive care unit. Crit Care Nurse 32(1):12–19
19. Baskin JL et al (2012) Thrombolytic therapy for central venous occlusion. Haematologica 97(5):641–650
20. Hadaway L (2006) Heparin locking for central venous catheters. JAVA 11(4)
21. NPSA (2008) Risks with intravenous heparin flush solutions. National Patient Safety Agency, London
22. Baranowski L (1993) Central venous access devices: current technologies, uses, and management strategies. J Intraven Nurs 16(3):167–194
23. Goodwin ML, Carlson I (1993) The peripherally inserted central catheter: a retrospective look at three years of insertions. J Intraven Nurs 16(2):92–103
24. Cummings-Winfield C, Mushani-Kanji T (2008) Restoring patency to central venous access devices. Clin J Oncol Nurs 12(6):925–934
25. Berreth M (2013) Flushing and locking part 2. INS Newsline, Jan/Feb 6–7
26. Hadaway L, Richardson D (2010) Needleless connectors: a primer on terminology. J Infus Nurs 33(1):22
27. Chernecky C, Macklin D, Casella L, Jarvis E (2009) Caring for patients with cancer through nursing knowledge of IV connectors. Clin J Oncol Nurs 13(6):630–633
28. Macklin D (2010) Catheter Management. Seminars in Oncology Nursing 26(2):113–120
29. Chernecky C and Waller J (2011) Comparative evaluation of five needless intravenous connectors. Journal of Advanced Nursing 67(7):1601–1613
30. Weinstein S, Plumer AL (2007) Plumer's principles and practice of intravenous therapy, 8th edn. Lippincott Williams and Wilkins, Philadelphia
31. Berger L (2000) The effects of positive pressure devices on catheter occlusions. J Vasc Access Devices 5(4):31–34
32. Lenhart C (2000) Prevention versus treatment of venous access device occlusions. J Vasc Access Devices 5(4):34–35
33. Rummel MA, Donnelly PJ, Fortenbaugh CC (2001) Clinical evaluation of a positive pressure device to prevent central venous catheter occlusion: results of a pilot study. Clin J Oncol Nurs 5(6):261–265
34. Solomon LR et al (2010) Observational study of need for thrombolytic therapy and incidence of bacteraemia using Taurolidine-citrate-heparin (TCH), Taurolidine-citrate (TC) and Heparin catheter locks in patient treated with haemodialysis. Am J Kidney Dis 55:1060–1068
35. Simon A, Ammann RA, Wiszniewsky G et al (2008) Taurolidine-citrate lock solution (TauroLock) significantly reduces CVAD-associated gram positive infections in pediatric cancer patients. BMC Infect Dis 8:102
36. Shah PS, Shah N (2007) Heparin bonded catheters for prolonging the patency of central venous catheters in children. Cochrane Database Syst Rev 2007(4):CD005983. doi:10.1002/14651858.CD005983.pub2
37. Couban S, Goodyear M, Burnell M et al (2005) Randomized placebo-controlled study of low-dose warfarin for the prevention of central venous catheter-associated thrombosis in patients with cancer. J Clin Oncol 23(18):4063–4069
38. Young AM, Begum G, Billingham LJ et al (2005) WARP: a multi-centre prospective randomised controlled trial (RCT) of thrombosis prophylaxis with warfarin in cancer patients with central venous catheters (CVCs). Abstract 8804. J Clin Oncol 23(16S)
39. Bishop L, Dougherty L, Bodenham A et al (2007) The British Committee for Standards in Haematology guidelines. Int J Haematol 29:261–278
40. Camp-Sorrell D, Cope DG, Oncology Nursing Society (2004) Access device guidelines: recommendations for nursing practice and education, 2nd edn. Oncology Nursing Society, Pittsburgh

41. Gorski L, Perucca R, Hunter M (2010) Central venous access devices: care, maintenance, and potential problems. In: Alexander M, Corrigan A, Gorski L et al (eds) Infusion nursing: an evidence-based approach, 3rd edn. Saunders/Elsevier, St Louis, pp 495–515
42. Gabriel J (2008) Long-term central venous access. In: Dougherty L, Lamb J (eds) Intravenous therapy in nursing practice, 2nd edn. Wiley Blackwell, Oxford
43. McKnight S (2004) Nurses guide to understanding and treating thrombotic occlusions of CVADs. Med Surg 13(6):377–382
44. Stewart D (2001) The percussion technique for restoring patency to central venous catheters. Care Crit Ill 17(3):106–107
45. Ponec D, Irwin D, Haire WD et al (2001) Recombinant tissue plasminogen activator (alteplase) for restoration of flow in occluded central venous access devices: a double-blind placebo-controlled trial. The cardiovascular thrombolytic to open occluded lines (COOL) efficacy trial. J Vasc Interv Radiol 12(8):951–955
46. Deitcher SR, Fesen MR, Kiproff PM et al (2002) Safety and efficacy of alteplase for restoring function in occluded central venous catheters: results of the cardiovascular thrombolytic to open occluded lines trial. J Clin Oncol 20(1):317–324
47. Timoney JP, Malkin MG, Leone DM et al (2002) Safe and cost effective use of alteplase for the clearance of occluded central venous access devices. J Clin Oncol 20(7):1918–1922
48. Van Miert C, Hill R, Jones L (2011) Interventions for restoring patency of occluded central venous catheter lumens. Cochrane Database Syst Rev 2012(4):CD007119. doi:10.1002/14651858.CD007119.pub2
49. Drewett SR (2009) Removal of central venous access devices. In: Hamilton H, Bodenham A (eds) Central venous catheters. Wiley-Blackwell, Chichester, pp 238–248
50. Ingle RJ (1995) Rare complications of vascular access devices. Semin Oncol Nurs 11(3):184–193
51. Andris DA, Krzywda EA (1997) Catheter pinch off syndrome: recognition and management. J Intraven Nurs 20(5):233–237
52. Hadaway L (1998) Catheter connection… are large syringes necessary? J Vasc Access Devices 3(3):40–41
53. Conn C (1993) The importance of syringe size when using an implanted vascular access device. J Vasc Access Netw 3(1):11–18
54. Reed T, Philips S (1996) Management of central venous catheters occlusion and repairs. J Intraven Nurs 19:289–294
55. Hadaway L (1998) Major thrombotic and non thrombotic complications: loss of patency. J Infus Nurs 1(5S):S143–S160

Clinical Problems Associated with the Use of Peripheral Venous Approaches: Infections

9

Giancarlo Scoppettuolo

9.1 Introduction

The rediscovery and widespread use of peripherally inserted central catheters (PICCs) is one of the most important innovations in the field of vascular access in recent years, including the application of ultrasound guidance for catheter insertion [1] and, in more recent years, the location of the correct position of the catheter's tip using the intracavitary EKG technique [2].

At present, PICCs are constantly expanding, and every year the number of devices that are inserted in both inpatients and outpatients increases. This is certainly due to the easy insertion and safety of the device, often performed by nurses or nursing teams; to the extremely low rate of complications, both immediate and late; to the multiple possibilities of use (thanks to the availability of new materials such as third generation polyurethanes and in particular the power-injectable polyurethane), from the infusion needs of patients admitted to acute wards or in the ICU up to chemotherapy and parenteral nutrition at home; and to clear cost-effectiveness.

Currently almost all PICCs over the world are inserted with ultrasound guidance.

In the last century, PICCs were placed without the use of the ultrasound system, exclusively in visible and/or palpable veins. This not only limited the insertions but made it possible to insert these devices only in the antecubital area or – but quite exceptionally – in the superficial veins of the forearm or arm. The insertion in the antecubital area, besides being particularly inconvenient for patients, implied an unacceptable (up to 30 %) rate of complications (dislocations, kinks, mechanical injuries, infections, thrombosis) basically due to the bending movement of the forearm on the arm.

G. Scoppettuolo, MD
Department of Infectious Disease, Catholic University,
L.go Gemelli, 8, 00168 Rome, Italy
e-mail: g.scoppettuolo@rm.unicatt.it

S. Sandrucci, B. Mussa (eds.), *Peripherally Inserted Central Venous Catheters*,
DOI 10.1007/978-88-470-5665-7_9, © Springer-Verlag Italia 2014

The spread of ultrasound guidance as gold standard for positioning has radically changed the history of vascular access in terms of eliminating complications and improving the success rates of the maneuver [3].

This was especially true for PICCs.

Since the beginning of this century, virtually all PICCs have been inserted using this technique, and the results of the insertions have dramatically changed.

The ultrasound guidance allows the cannulation of the arm's deep veins (especially basilic and brachial veins), using a modified Seldinger technique (venipuncture with a small-bore needle, inserting a guidewire through the needle and then removing the needle itself, removing the guidance and dilator, inserting the catheter through the introducer). With this technique, the failure rate as well as potential complications at the time of insertion is almost zero. Above all, the exit site is located in an area defined by some American authors as the "green zone" [4], which is the middle arm, midway between the elbow and the armpit.

The possibility of an exit site in that area, besides determining a much greater comfort for the patient, made it possible to substantially reduce the rate of late complications in terms of infections, thrombosis, dislocations, etc.

The exit site in the middle of the arm has many advantages, especially in relation to the possibilities of developing an infection: (1) it is practically not influenced by movement of the forearm on the arm; (2) it is located in an area with low bacterial colonization (10^2 CFU/mm^2); (3) it represents a perfect area for a stable and lasting medication and enables fixing the catheter appropriately; and (4) it is far from areas potentially capable of determining a colonization of the catheter, such as the patient's mouth or nose or a possible tracheostomy, through contaminated secretions often also with multiresistant microorganisms.

9.2 PICC-Related Infection Pathogenesis

To fully understand the strategies for preventing bloodstream infections related to PICC – as well as for each type of central venous catheter – it is important to remember the pathogenesis of colonization, which constitutes the first and essential moment for the subsequent development of a clinically significant infection.

A PICC, like any other central venous catheter, can be colonized by microorganisms primarily through two mechanisms: extraluminal and intraluminal [5] (Fig. 9.1).

The extraluminal colonization basically occurs when the microorganisms present in the superficial and deeper layers of a patient's skin and on unwashed or badly washed hands of health professionals or people who take care of the catheter migration. They attach to the outer surface of the catheter, the first outer section, then on the section located in the subcutaneous tissue, and on the section inside the blood vessel. As a result, extraluminal prevention of colonization will be performed effectively through mechanisms aimed at lowering the microbial load present on the patient's skin and on the hands of people that assist him/her and to protect the catheter insertion site. In other words, washing hands, proper skin antisepsis at the time of insertion and after insertion, proper dressing technique of the catheter exit site.

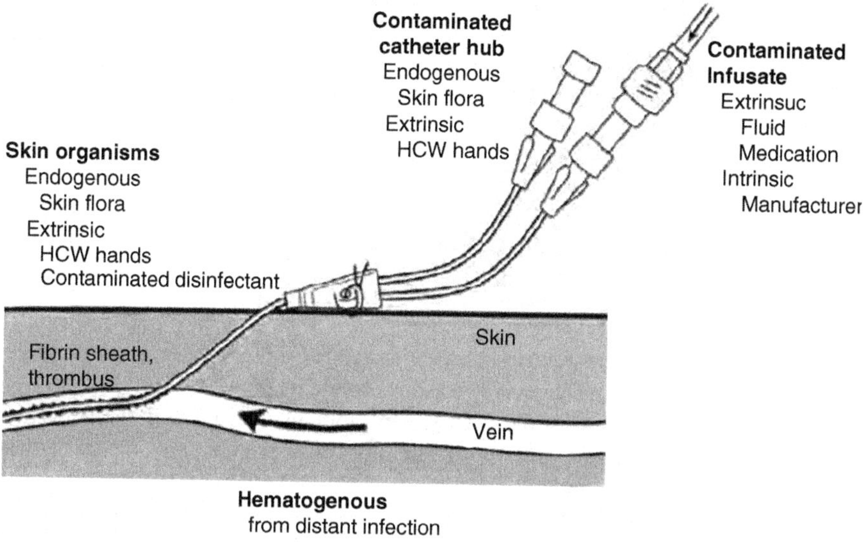

Fig. 9.1 Pathogenesis of extra- and intraluminal colonization (Reproduced with permission from [5])

Colonization occurs intraluminally when microorganisms present at the hub of the catheter, the injectable ports, connectors, and infusion lines are injected into the catheter during infusion. This happens when the hands of the person making the infusion are not properly washed, when the access to the catheter is done without adequate disinfection of the catheter hub (including the needle-free connectors), and when the infusion lines (and possibly needle-free connectors, if used) are not replaced adequately.

Regarding PICCs, the two ways of catheter colonization and infection certainly have a different impact.

With regard to the extraluminal colonization, it is considered that PICCs – more than any other type of vascular access – have an exit site that is perfect for dressing, in an area with relatively low spontaneous colonization. Besides that, in most care settings, there is a good adherence to proper medication techniques. Another factor to consider is the length of the catheter, which is usually twice or more than any other central venous access. This makes the route that organisms must go through particularly long to reach colonizing the catheter tip and then triggering a clinically relevant infection.

For these reasons, the extraluminal colonization is considered secondary for PICCs and certainly less important than the intraluminal route.

The intraluminal colonization, as mentioned, is mainly due to poor management of the hub and the infusion lines and in particular to a lack of or inadequate disinfection of the hub when connecting the infusion line. In most hospitals facing the increased awareness of the importance in dressing the exit site and a good adherence to a proper technique, compliance to a proper disinfection of the hub is very low.

This is also evidenced by the increase in Gram-negative organisms and fungi as etiologic agents of central venous catheter bloodstream infections.

The different impacts of the extra- and intraluminal colonization as triggering mechanisms of infections related to the PICC would also be reflected in the fact that, as we will see later, the PICCs implanted in outpatients with intermittent use of the catheter have an infection rate lower than the PICCs used in inpatients, where access to hubs occur several times daily.

9.3   Epidemiology

The analysis of the papers published on PICC-related infections – especially meta-analysis – is very difficult for several reasons.

First, before 2000s most of the PICCs were implanted without ultrasound guidance and in the antecubital area, with infection rates significantly different than would have happened recently.

Another factor to take into consideration is that the use of PICC in hospitalized patients and in nonhospitalized patients is considerably different regarding the risk of infections.

Finally, only in recent times, bundles for prevention of PICC-related infections have been applied in clinical practice.

Generally, infection rates are reported for hospitalized patients ranging from 0 to 6.5 BSI per 1,000 catheter days, with a very wide variability.

In a retrospective study of Lam et al. out of 135 PICC in hospitalized patients, the rate of BSI reported was 1.6 per 1,000 catheter days [6].

Chait et al. reported a bloodstream infection rate of 2.1 per 1,000 PICC catheter days implanted in children [7].

Another retrospective study by Cowl et al. in patients receiving parenteral nutrition at home does not report BSI related to PICCs [8].

In a prospective study, PICCs inserted in 111 children hospitalized for total parenteral nutrition, Yeung et al. reported a rate of 6.4 BSI per 1,000 catheter days [9].

A similar rate of infection has been reported in a small retrospective study on pregnant women [10].

A PICC study in hematologic patients by Hunter et al. documented a rate of 2.2 per 1,000 catheter days [11].

In one of the works investigated extensively, although with the limitations just mentioned, the rate of PICC infection was performed prospectively in two randomized trials to test the efficacy in the prevention of bloodstream infections of chlorhexidine-impregnated sponges and skin antisepsis with chlorhexidine. The work considered 115 patients with 251 PICCs, with an average catheterization time of 11.3 days and for a total of 2,832 catheter days. Forty-two percent of patients were in intensive care. A rate of PICC-related bloodstream infections equal to 2.1 per 1,000 catheter days was found [12].

In the same study, besides considering the patients included in the two randomized trials and followed prospectively, a literature review that included 33 studies

(19 on children and 14 on adults) was performed. The average rate of PICC-related bloodstream infections emerged from the audit was just 2.1 per 1,000 catheter days (1.9 for adults and 2.2 for children), similar to that observed prospectively.

The authors conclude that the average rate of PICC-related bloodstream infections is comparable to that of short-term non-tunneled CVC, representing approximately 2.3 per 1,000 catheter days, higher than the long-term tunneled CVCs (1.0 per 1,000 catheter days) and higher than that of PICCs used in outpatients.

Similarly, but emphasizing a clear difference between patients hospitalized and not, Maki, in a meta-analysis that appeared in 2006, reported an infection rate of 2.1 for PICCs used in hospitalized patients and 1.1 for PICCs used in outpatients. In the same study, the average rate of short-term non-tunneled CVC infection was measured in 2.7 and long-term tunneled CVC in 1.1 [13].

Raiy et al. conducted a prospective comparative study of central venous catheters (CVC) and PICC in patients admitted to non-intensive care units. 638 CVC and 622 PICC were included in the study. Catheter-related bloodstream infection rates observed were similar, respectively, 2.4 and 2.3 BSI per 1,000 catheter days. The interesting finding of the study is that the average time for PICC infection is significantly longer than the CVC (23 vs.13 days) [14].

In another prospective study in a surgical intensive care unit, the PICC infection rate was considerably lower than that of CVC (2.2 vs. 6.0 BSI per 1,000 catheter days) [15].

Bellesi et al. reported a very low rate of BSI in patients undergoing autologous bone marrow transplantation. Sixty-six PICCs were included in the study inserted in 57 patients, with an overall 1.236 catheter days. The bloodstream infection rate was 1.5 per 1,000 catheter days [16].

More recently, Chopra et al. performed a systematic review and meta-analysis on the risk of bloodstream infections associated with PICCs compared with central venous catheters in adults. Authors found that PICCs were associated with a lower risk of bloodstream infections than central venous catheters in outpatients. Moreover, hospitalized patients who underwent PICC placement experienced similar risk of bloodstream infections than patients with central venous catheters and a tenfold greater risk than outpatients with PICCs [17].

There are also a number of very recent studies that are all characterized by some common factors: ultrasound guidance insertion and insertion and care bundles including some important points of the current international recommendations (use of 2 % chlorhexidine, sutureless devices, transparent semipermeable dressings, etc.). All these studies report extremely low BSI rates, even zero.

In contrast, in the studies reported above, the insertion in most cases was not done with ultrasound guidance, or this kind of information was not reported. Similarly, the management methods used are never reported.

The first of these studies was published by Harnage et al., who got a sustained absence of PICC-related bloodstream infections by using a bundle insertion and management in a community-based hospital [18].

Cotogni et al. reported prospective data on four types of central venous catheters in cancer patients on home parenteral nutrition. Two hundred and forty-nine vascular accesses were studied, for a total of 51,308 catheter days. Sixty-five PICCs for a total of 11,504 catheter days were included in the study. The PICC-related bloodstream infection rate was zero. An interesting finding of the study is the statistically significant association between the use of ultrasound and sutureless devices for the stabilization of the catheter and the absence of bloodstream infections [19].

Even Botella-Carretero et al. reported a zero rate of BSI in 48 PICCs patients used in home parenteral nutrition [20].

Pittiruti et al. reported an infection rate of zero for 89 PICC power-injectables used in adult and pediatric intensive care unit [21].

Scoppettuolo et al. conducted a case-control study to test the effectiveness of an insertion and maintenance bundle for preventing PICC-related bloodstream infections. The study included 120 patients who applied the bundle and 360 controls not subjected to the bundle. The rate of BSI was equal to zero in the study group while in the control group was equal to 2.66 BSI per 1,000 catheter days [22].

Moraza-Dulanto et al. report an experience of 165 PICCs placed in oncoematologic patients, with an infection rate very close to zero (0.06 per 1,000 catheter days) [23].

9.4   Prevention

Until a few years ago, the goal of central line-associated bloodstream infection prevention (CLABSI) was their reduction below a certain benchmark value. Over recent years, however, the possibility of zeroing CLABSI was suggested. According to the philosophy of the so-called Targeting Zero [21] by the Association for Professionals in Infection Control and Epidemiology (APIC), mind-changing was necessary, with reference to nosocomial infections in general and CLABSI in particular. Starting from the idea that complications, and therefore infections, are not inevitable, but rather are caused by incorrect operator behavior, the new goal of prevention strategies and campaigns was zeroing CLABSI and not reducing them. This concept is expressed clearly by the CDC guidelines of 2011, indicating that zeroing CLABSI is the objective of prevention from all care areas or, at worst, their reduction to the lowest possible value [24].

Over the years, several papers have shown that targeting zero is a possible result. The most famous of these is the experience gained in 108 ICUs in Michigan, which zeroed catheter-related infections, maintaining this result for a long period of time. The instrument that resulted in eliminating CLABSI in the Michigan Keystone Project was the "bundle." The bundle is the implementation of a number of strong indications derived from the guidelines, generally from four to eight, which, if applied simultaneously by all operators and for all patients, ensures the best possible outcome. The bundle must be spread and used by all operators, and its application must be verified by specially designed checklists. The bundle applied in ICUs in Michigan was composed of five simple steps, easy to remember, easy to apply, and low cost: hand washing, use of maximal barrier precautions when inserting the catheter, rational choice of the catheter insertion site, use of chlorhexidine for skin

Table 9.1 GAVeCeLT bundle for PICC-related bloodstream infection prevention

Hand hygiene
Maximal sterile barrier precautions during PICC insertion
Ultrasound-guided insertion
Use of 2 % chlorhexidine for skin antisepsis before insertion and for continuous or discontinuous exit site's antisepsis during management and for disinfection of catheter's hub or needlefree connectors
Use of "sutureless devices" for catheter's securement
Use of transparent dressing
Prompt removal of unnecessary PICCs

antisepsis, and daily review of the catheter need, with immediate removal when it is no longer essential [25].

As can be seen, this bundle, being designed for short-term catheters, is more about the time of insertion than for management. Other bundles (e.g., GAVeCeLT, Italian Group for the Study of Long-Term Vascular Access), designed for medium-term catheters, take into account both the time of insertion and that of post-insertion care [22] (Table 9.1).

In a recent supplement of *Annals of Internal Medicine* devoted to the practices to be implemented as soon as possible for the safety of the patient, the use of bundles that include a checklist for the prevention of CLABSI is considered among the actions that should be "strongly encouraged" [26].

As previously mentioned, PICC features of insertion and management make them the perfect vascular catheters for the prevention of infection, as demonstrated by a lot of previously reported studies, where the rate of PICC-related bloodstream infections is equal to zero.

Currently, an effective prevention of CLABSI related to PICCs, like those related to other types of central venous catheters, should provide for the implementation of behavioral strategies and technological strategies to be applied prior to insertion of the catheter, upon insertion, and subsequently, during management [24, 27–29].

Such strategies should preferably be "bundled," and their application must be verified by an appropriate checklist.

Prior to insertion of the catheter, it is important that trained personnel carefully choose the best type of access for each individual patient, taking into account the different risk of infection related to different types of venous access.

The time of insertion, often overlooked in the past, has a crucial importance in the prevention of CLABSI and is done properly by applying an aseptic technique; using maximal barrier precautions; using chlorhexidine for skin antisepsis; using ultrasound guidance, not only to avoid the mechanical complications but also and especially infectious ones; and carefully choosing, above all, the catheter insertion site and the catheter implantation technique.

The third moment of CLABSI prevention is the proper management of the catheter. Management is an essential time because it virtually affects the entire life of the catheter and is directly responsible for the lives of the catheter. The administration of the therapy safely, without complications potentially fatal or that otherwise,

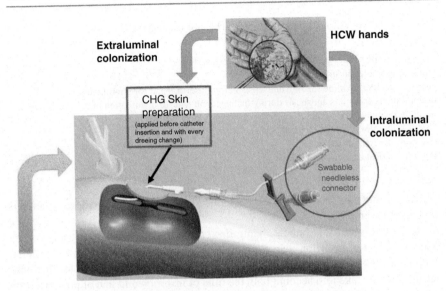

Fig. 9.2 Prevention of extra- and intraluminal colonization

in the best situations, determines the need for hospitalization, additional costs, and deterioration of the patient's quality of life. The insertion of a catheter is certainly important; it represents a very small part of the life of a catheter, where the management represents the main part.

Proper management of a catheter is accomplished primarily through proper care of the exit site and proper access to the infusion lines and the correct replacement of these [30] (Fig. 9.2).

Below there is a list of behavioral and technological strategies useful for the prevention of CLABSI associated with central venous catheters, including PICC.

9.4.1 Behavioral Strategies

9.4.1.1 Education
One of the most effective tools indicated by the guidelines for the prevention of CLABSI is the education of the people involved in the insertion and management of vascular catheters and on the CLABSI risk and strategies for infection prevention in general. The correct insertion procedures (including the use of the ultrasound guidance) and, above all, on proper management procedures, with the ability to perform – for health professionals but also and especially for caregivers – an adequate training process [24, 27–29].

Education must be subjected to periodic updates and constant verification in terms of knowledge, adherence, and application, using specially developed tools such as checklists [28].

Even for patients who use PICCs at home, education is a crucial aspect for CLABSI prevention.

The education and training process for the patient with PICCs and for the caregiver, made by an expert, is expected to begin in the hospital before discharge and then continues on the territory. The aim of providing information is to learn the basic techniques for proper management of the PICC, in order to be autonomous in the maneuver and to minimize complications. Another purpose of education and training should be represented by clear guidance on the symptoms and warning signs of complications, when they have already occurred and when to ask for assistance [31].

Training can be performed effectively with different interventions ranging from practical demonstrations of procedures by personnel experienced in the delivery of written material (see ASPEN Handbook) or the use of DVDs, online videos, tutorials, etc. [32].

It is also important to remember the particular context in which the process of education takes place for outpatients: patients and their families whose primary concern is the diagnosis for which a PICC is required and the awareness to start managing a very important device for survival but also its potential danger.

Several studies have documented the effectiveness of education and training in the prevention of complications. Back in 1994, Moukarzel et al. [33] showed that in a pediatric population performing home parenteral nutrition, one of the most important predictors of the catheter longevity and a low rate of infectious complications was represented by adequate training of family members.

Finally, an educational strategy for outpatients that has been very successful in recent years and is proving to be very effective is the creation of websites, especially for patients applying home parenteral nutrition and for their families and cancer patients [34].

9.4.1.2 Hand Washing

Hand washing is clearly the most effective and economical tool for the prevention of health-care-associated infections and, in particular, of CLABSI. Besides health-care professionals, the patient and the caregiver should be instructed on the importance of hand washing and the proper technique to do it, either with soap and water or even better with more effective alcohol-based gel, faster and less damaging to the skin.

Hands should be washed before and after each contact with the patient and with the patient's catheter (at the time of the insertion, palpation of the exit site, dressing change, access to the infusion line, replacement or repair).

The problems that mainly hinder the poor implementation of hand hygiene are the lack of information on the importance of the procedure and technique, low adherence (though higher in patients and caregivers, as well as among nurses compared to physicians), and poor diffusion mechanisms to control the adherence [23, 27–29, 35].

9.4.1.3 Use of Checklist

The use of a checklist is recommended by SHEA/IDSA guidelines to verify adherence of health-care workers to aseptic techniques during insertion and maintenance of PICCs in a very effective way. A nurse should preferably complete the checklist other than inserts or take care of the PICC [28].

9.4.2   Technological Strategies

9.4.2.1 Ultrasound Guidance Insertion

The use of ultrasound guidance is now the gold standard for the insertion of any CVC. The ultrasound system increases the success of the maneuver at the first attempt; significantly reduces the number of attempts to venipuncture; minimizes significant mechanical complications such as pneumothorax, hemothorax, and arterial puncture; and reduces the time needed for insertion and associated costs.

The ultrasound guidance insertion is also effective in reducing CLABSI. This is achieved through various mechanisms. First, limit the number of needle punctures through the skin before puncture of the vein effectively allows a lower colonization of the needle that passes through the deep structures of the skin, which, as is known, cannot be subjected to a totally effective antisepsis. The possibility, then, to be able to puncture the vein at the first attempt reduces the possibility of forming hematomas, which is a real breeding ground for microorganisms.

The use of ultrasound guidance is now recommended by the main international guidelines for the prevention of CRBSI as an effective tool [3, 24, 27, 29].

As pointed out by the CDC guidelines and other more recent guidelines, the people using ultrasound must receive appropriate training [3, 24, 36].

9.4.2.2 Two Percent Chlorhexidine

Chlorhexidine is a topical antiseptic solution that has been used worldwide since 1954, with an excellent safety profile and efficacy in both adults and children.

Chlorhexidine is today one of the most effective tools for the prevention of hospital-acquired infections in general, and especially clearly and amply demonstrated, for CRBSI. Over the past 20 years, numerous studies have tried to show what was the best antiseptic to the skin before inserting a CVC, during dressing changes, and during any manipulation of the catheter. On the basis of current and very clear evidence from 2007 onwards – the year in which EPIC2 guidelines were published – chlorhexidine is the preferred antiseptic for the prevention of CLABSI, preferred to jodopovidone and alcohol. Chlorhexidine is bactericidal; it has a very broad spectrum; it is quickly active (30 s after application, compared to 120 s of povidone iodine); it has a prolonged antimicrobial effect; and it is in synergy with alcohol and is not inactivated by blood or other body fluids, unlike jodopovidone.

Currently all of the guidelines for the prevention of CLABSI highlight the greater effectiveness of chlorhexidine compared to povidone iodine and alcohol and recommend it as an antiseptic at the time of catheter insertion and the subsequent continuous or discontinuous antisepsis of the exit site during dressing [24, 27–29].

The type of chlorhexidine to be chosen is a solution of chlorhexidine gluconate 2 % preferably in isopropyl alcohol of 70 % (isopropyl alcohol is not detrimental to the polyurethane of which most catheters are composed, unlike ethyl alcohol), preferably colored solution, and preferably in small packs or, better, applicators for single patient use.

9.4.2.3 Chlorhexidine-Impregnated Sponges

For several years, polyurethane impregnated sponges were introduced in the market enabling a sustained release of chlorhexidine gluconate at 2 % (24 h a day for 7 days) applied at the catheter exit site and replaced every 7 days to prevent colonization. Given the effectiveness of chlorhexidine as an antiseptic, a device such as the one described above is certainly reasonable. On the other hand, numerous works and some meta-analysis have demonstrated clearly that these sponges are able to prevent exit site colonization, catheter tip colonization, and clinically more relevant CLABSI. Currently the use of these sponges is recommended by the SHEA/IDSA guidelines and CDC but with restrictions and limited to certain categories of patients at high risk of developing CLABSI or serious consequences as a result of CLABSI (e.g., heart valve wearers or vascular prosthesis) or in patients who, having already had repeated CLABSI, have no more options for repositioning a CVC [27–29].

9.4.2.4 Sutureless Devices

Until a few years ago, the standard for catheter stabilization was represented by stitches, with a considerable series of disadvantages that increase the risk of infection and thrombosis: interrupting the integrity of the skin around the exit site; early and persistent bacterial colonization; non optimal attachment of the catheter, resulting in "in and out" movement of the same; patient discomfort; and risk of operator accidental puncture when suturing [24, 27].

In recent years, devices called "sutureless" were designed to fix catheters, consisting of a band aid, which contains an implantation for the catheter wings on top. Several papers, especially on PICCs, have shown that the sutureless devices stabilize the catheters safely and effectively, not compromising the integrity of the skin; they avoid movements of the catheter due to the effective stabilization; they reduce bacterial colonization around the exit site, being replaced every 7 days; and they are greatly appreciated by patients and operators (including the elimination of the accidental puncture risk).

9.4.2.5 Proper Dressing of Exit Site

As mentioned previously, proper medication is essential in the prevention of extraluminal catheter colonization and is one of two crucial points during the management of a central venous catheter [24, 27–29].

Proper dressing is carried out via an aseptic technique, using an effective antiseptic (chlorhexidine 2 %) and choosing an appropriate dressing.

The majority of current guidelines recommend gauze and tape medications as well as transparent semipermeable dressings to protect the exit site without preferences, with gauze and tape requiring replacement every 48 h and transparent dressings every 7 days, with the foresight of immediate change for both if they are dirty, wet, or loose.

Only the EPIC2 guidelines and ESPEN guidelines identify semipermeable transparent dressings as preferable, with the following advantages: visibility of the insertion site; better stabilization of the catheter, with reduced "in and out" movements; protection from secretions; and possibility of replacing every 7 days [27, 29].

Fig. 9.3 Semipermeable transparent dressing and chlorhexidine-impregnated sponge to protect exit site

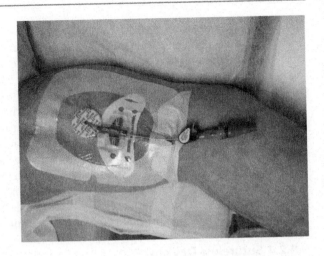

A new protection strategy of the PICC exit site especially at the time of insertion is represented by the use of glue. In fact, using this method is effective in preventing bleeding after PICC insertion, as well as in preventing dislocation through better stabilization of the device. The glue used at the time of implantation as a seal for the protection of the exit site could also, by analogy to the use of the same in other areas of surgery, prevent bacterial colonization [37] (Fig. 9.3).

9.4.2.6 Access Technique to the Infusion Line (Including Disinfection of Hubs and Needle-Free Connectors) and Replacement of Infusion Lines

The second essential point in the management of a PICC after dressing is the access technique to the infusion line and the frequency of changing infusion lines. As dressing prevents the extraluminal catheter colonization, so a proper aseptic technique to access the catheter ensures the prevention of intraluminal colonization. Today, in all likelihood, the majority of CLABSI recognizes a pathogenetic mechanism due to poor adherence to the disinfection of the catheter access points prior to use.

Each access point to the catheter (catheter hub, connectors, stopcocks, etc.) must be thoroughly disinfected before infusion.

At the moment, there is not enough data to give strong and definitive indications on proper disinfection technique of catheters hubs.

Guidelines recommend vigorously scrubbing the access of a catheter with chlorhexidine, povidone iodine, or alcohol, not specifying the time of contact, which, according to some papers and expert opinions, should be around 15 s [38].

PICCs are very often closed by needle-free connectors (NFC). Such devices were introduced at the beginning of the 1990s in order to avoid the risk of accidental needle injuries, allowing access to the infusion system without the use of needles. A second effect regards the protection of the catheter occlusions, since the NFCs are based on an internal mechanisms that determine a negative, neutral, or positive displacement resulting in a minimum backflow of blood into the catheter upon disconnection (negative displacement), no backflow (neutral displacement), or leaking from the catheter of a small quantity of solution accumulated in a reservoir of the NFC to "wash" the catheter. In addition, the various NFC models available on the market are highly variable with regard to the regularity of the external surface, the fixing mechanism of the infusion line (which can be "luer lock" or simply pressure inserted by passing through a split septum), the regularity of flow inside, and transparent design or not. Since the NFC is a part to be disinfected before connecting the line, in addition to the two effects mentioned above, they are directly involved in the possibility to determine the colonization of the catheter and subsequent CLABSI. It is easily understood, then, that the more the external surface and septum is smooth, all the more simple shall it be to disinfect them, as the more regular and visible is the internal flow, the lower the risk of colonization [39, 40].

There are many studies on NFCs, often conflicting, whereby the guidelines provide few messages. First, as every catheter entry point, the NFCs should be disinfected before use in the way described above; they must be replaced with the infusion line, but not more frequently than every 72 h; they must be compatible with the infusion system; and they should not involve positive displacement, due to increased risk of infection [24].

Infusion lines must be replaced every 24 h if they have been used to infuse blood or blood products or solutions containing lipids. In case of continuous infusions that do not include the above substances, infusion lines should be replaced not more frequently than every 96 h but at least every 7 days [24, 27–29].

References

1. Simcock L (2008) No going back: advantages of ultrasound-guided upper arm PICC placement. JAVA 13(4):191–197
2. Pittiruti M, La Greca A, Scoppettuolo G (2011) The electrocardiographic method for positioning the tip of central venous catheters. J Vasc Access 12(4):280–291
3. Lamperti M, Bodenham AR, Pittiruti M et al (2012) International evidence-based recommendations on ultrasound-guided vascular access. Intensive Care Med 38(7):1105–1117
4. Dawson RB (2011) PICC Zone Insertion Method™ (ZIM™): a systematic approach to determine the ideal insertion site for PICCs in the upper arm. JAVA 16(3):156–165
5. Crnich CY, Maki DG (2002) The promise of novel technology for the prevention of intravascular device-related bloodstream infections. Pathogenesis and short-term device. Clin Infect Dis 34(9):1232–1242
6. Lam S, Scannell R, Roessler D et al (1994) Peripherally inserted central catheters in an acute-care hospital. Arch Intern Med 154:1833–1837
7. Chait PG, Ingram J, Phillips-Gordon C et al (1995) Peripherally inserted central catheters in children. Radiology 197:775–778
8. Cowl CT, Weinstock JV, Al-Jurf A et al (2000) Complications and cost associated with parenteral nutrition delivered to hospitalized patients through either subclavian or peripherally inserted central catheters. Clin Nutr 19:237–243
9. Yeung CY, Lee HC, Huang FY et al (1998) Sepsis during total parenteral nutrition: exploration of risk factors and determination of the effectiveness of peripherally inserted central venous catheters. Pediatr Infect Dis J 17:135–142
10. Ogura JM, Francois KE, Perlow JH et al (2003) Complications associated with peripherally inserted central catheter use during pregnancy. Am J Obstet Gynecol 188:1223–1225

11. Harter C, Ostendorf T, Bach A et al (2003) Peripherally inserted central venous catheters for autologous blood progenitor cell transplantation in patients with haematological malignancies. Support Care Cancer 11:790–794
12. Safdar N, Maki DG (2005) Risk of catheter-related bloodstream infection with peripherally inserted central venous catheters used in adults patients. Chest 128:489–495
13. Maki DG, Kluger DK, Crnick CJ (2006) The risk of bloodstream infection in adults with different intravascular devices: a systematic review of 200 published prospective studies. Mayo Clin Proc 81(9):1159–1171
14. Al Raiy B, Fakih MG, Brvan-Nomides N et al (2010) Peripherally inserted central venous catheters in the acute care setting: a safe alternative to high risk short term central venous catheters. Am J Infect Control 38(2):149–153
15. Gunst M, Matsushima K, Vanek S et al (2012) Peripherally inserted central venous catheters may lower the incidence of catheter-related bloodstream infections in surgical intensive care units. Surg Infect (Larchmt) 12(4):279–282
16. Bellesi S, Chiusolo P, De Pascale G et al (2013) Peripherally inserted central venous catheters (PICCs) in the management of oncohematological patients submitted to autologous stem cell transplant. Support Care Cancer 21(2):531–535
17. Chopra V, O'Horo J, Rogers MAM et al (2013) The risk of bloodstream infection associate with peripherally inserted central catheters compared with central venous catheters in adults: a systematic review and meta-analysis. Infect Control Hosp Epidemiol 34(9):908–918
18. Harnage SA (2007) Achieving zero catheter related bloodstream infections: 15 months success in a community based medical center. JAVA 12(4):218–225
19. Cotogni P, Pittiruti M, Barbero C et al (2013) Catheter-related complications in cancer patients on home parenteral nutrition: a prospective study of over 51.000 catheter days. JPEN J Parenter Enteral Nutr 37(3):375–383
20. Botella-Carretero J, Carrero C, Guerra E et al (2013) Role of peripherally inserted central catheters in home parenteral nutrition: a 5-year prospective study. JPEN J Parenter Enteral Nutr 37(4):544–549
21. Pittiruti M, Brutti A, Celentano D et al (2012) Clinical experience with power-injectable PICCs in intensive care patients. Crit Care 16(1):R21
22. Scoppettuolo G, Dolcetti L, Taraschi C et al (2011) Targeting Zero CLABSI in patients with PICC lines: a case-control study. Poster #37, Association for Vascular Access annual scientific meeting, San José, 3–6 Oct 2011
23. Association for Professional in Infection Control and Epidemiology (APIC). http://utility.apic.org/AM/CM/ContentDisplay.cfm?ContentFileID=11707. Accessed 01.10.2013
24. O'Grady NP, Alexander M, Burns LA et al (2011) Guidelines for the prevention of intravascular catheter-related infections. Clin Infect Dis 2011 52(9):e162–e193
25. Pronovost P, Needham D, Berenholtz S et al (2006) An intervention to decrease catheter-related bloodstream infections in the ICU. N Engl J Med 355(26):2725–2732
26. Shekelle PG, Pronovost PJ, Wachter RM et al (2013) The Top Patient Safety Strategies that can be encouraged for adoption now. Ann Intern Med 158:365–368
27. Pittiruti M, Hamilton H, Biffi R et al (2009) ESPEN guidelines on parenteral nutrition. Clin Nutr 28:365–377
28. Marshall J, Mermel LA, Classen D et al (2008) Strategies to prevent central line-associated bloodstream infections in acute care hospital. Infect Control Hosp Epidemiol 29:S22–S30
29. Pratt RJ, Pellowe CM, Wilson JA et al (2007) EPIC2: national evidence-based guidelines for preventing healthcare-associated infections in NHS hospitals in England. J Hosp Infect 65:S1–S64
30. Ryder M (2006) Evidence-based practice in the management of vascular access devices for home parenteral nutrition therapy. JPEN J Parenter Enteral Nutr 30:S82–S93
31. Kumpf VJ, Tillman EM (2012) Home parenteral nutrition: safe transition from hospital to home. Nutr Clin Pract 27:749–757
32. Gifford H, DeLegge M, Epperson LA (2010) Education methods and techniques for training home parenteral nutrition patients. Nutr Clin Pract 25:443–450

33. Moukarzel AA, Haddad I, Ament ME et al (1994) 230 patients years of experience with long-term parenteral nutrition in childhood: natural history and life of central venous catheters. J Pediatr Surg 29:1323–1327

34. Fitzgerald SA, Macan Yadrich D, Wercowitch M et al (2011) Creating patient and education web sites. Design and content of the home parenteral nutrition family caregivers web sites. Comput Inform Nurs 29(11):637–645

35. World Health Organization (2009) WHO Guidelines on hand hygiene in health care

36. Moreau N, Lamperti M, Kelly LJ et al (2013) Evidence-based consensus on the insertion of central venous access devices: definition of minimal requirements for training. Br J Anaesth 110(3):347–356

37. Annetta MG, Pittiruti M, Scoppettuolo G et al (2013) Randomized clinical study on the efficacy of metallic powder vs. cyanoacrylate glue in sealing the exit site of peripherally inserted central catheters: preliminary results. Poster #81, Association for Vascular Access Annual Scientific Meeting, Nashville, 20–23 Sept 2013

38. Kaler W, Chinn R (2007) Successful disinfection of needleless access port: a matter of time and friction. JAVA 12(3):140–142

39. Hadaway L (2012) Needleless connectors for IV catheters. Am J Nurs 112(11):32–44

40. Btaiche IF, Kovacevich DS, Khalidi N et al (2011) The effects of needleless connectors on catheter-related bloodstream infections. Am J Infect Control 39(4):277–283

Clinical Problems Associated with the Use of Peripheral Venous Approaches in Clinical Practice: Thrombosis

10

Cristina Garrino

PICCs are becoming diffused because of their low risk of early complications, the possibility of nurse insertion, the simple management even at home, and the low rate of CVC-related infections, compared to other types of central venous access [1, 2]. Moreover, with rising health-care costs, the trend is to favor outpatient care, and in this perspective the need for long-term venous access, and PICCs in particular, is expected to further increase [3].

However, these devices are not as harmless as initially believed: with the widespread diffusion of PICCs, an increasing number of symptomatic upper limb deep vein thrombosis (DVT) has been observed [4, 5].

Venous thromboembolism is known to be an important complication in patients carrying a CVC [6, 7]; furthermore, it is one of the leading causes for death in this group of patients [8], and central venous catheters (CVCs) used for chemotherapy administration have recently been indicated as an additional risk for developing venous thrombosis [9, 10]. CVC-related deep vein thrombosis (DVT) represents the second cause for catheter removal, after infection, in cancer patients [11].

A misdiagnosed deep vein thrombosis can carry very serious consequences, varying between post-thrombotic syndrome and the not infrequent pulmonary thromboembolism [12–15]; in particular, the pulmonary thromboembolism rate in the case of upper limb CVC-related DVT is reported to be about 12–17 % [16]. Whether asymptomatic CVC-associated DVT has the same clinical relevance as symptomatic venous thrombosis remains to be determined.

In scientific literature, PICC-related venous thrombosis seems to have, depending on different studies, an incidence rate varying from 10 to 60 % of patients [17]. This variability is likely to be linked to heterogeneity of study design, patient population, diagnostic techniques, the type of catheter positioned, and the distinction between symptomatic and asymptomatic thrombosis. The majority of data now

C. Garrino
Dipartimento Chirurgia Oncologica,
Ospedale Molinette, Corso Bramante 88, Torino 10129, Italy
email: crigarr@hotmail.com

S. Sandrucci, B. Mussa (eds.), *Peripherally Inserted Central Venous Catheters*,
DOI 10.1007/978-88-470-5665-7_10, © Springer-Verlag Italia 2014

available is based on retrospective studies about symptomatic venous thrombosis [18, 19]; a few prospective studies mainly regarding the intensive care unit report an incidence of asymptomatic thrombosis between 27.5 and 58 % [20, 21], one study having been stopped for the unacceptable rate of thrombosis probably due to the dimension of the catheter (6 Fr triple lumen) [22].

10.1 Physiopathological Basis

A catheter-related thrombosis (CRDVT) is defined as a deep vein or large limb vein thrombosis developing in a vessel where a vascular catheter has been positioned.
A catheter-related thrombosis can be classified as follows [23]:

- Fibrin sheath (slim "film" of fibrin surrounding the catheter). In clinical practice, it is almost always diagnosed when it is localized on the tip, as it typically causes the so-called withdrawal occlusion, e.g., difficulty or impossibility to withdraw blood from the catheter due to a "valve effect" of the fibrin sheath on the catheter tip.
- Intraluminal clot (adherent to the catheter but not to the vessel wall).
- Mural thrombosis (clot surrounding the catheter and adhering to the vein wall, but not occupying the entire lumen of the vessel).
- Occlusive venous thrombosis (occupying the entire lumen of the vessel, therefore blocking blood flow).
  On this basis, CRDVT can be more or less symptomatic.

For that which concerns the risk factors of thrombosis, they are referred conventionally to as the so-called Virchow's triad (from Rudolf Virchow, a German pathologist who first hypothesized in 1875 the mechanism of thrombus pathogenesis): stasis, vascular injury, and hypercoagulability.

Central venous catheters impact fundamentally on two of them, namely, vascular injury and stasis: in particular, PICCs are inserted into smaller veins than classic CVCs, leading to a more evident blood flow reduction ("stasis"). In an experimental model, reported a 60 % flow reduction in a 4 mm tube filled with a circulating blood-simulating solution and containing a 4 Fr wire and a 58 % flow reduction in a 5 mm tube containing a 5 Fr wire [24].

The endovascular catheter also acts as a cause of endothelial damage, both at the entry point into the vein and at the tip, with a "scrubbing" effect on the endothelial surface. Endothelial injury predisposes thrombus formation through three mechanisms: platelet activators, such as exposed subendothelial collagen, which promote platelet adhesion to the damaged site; tissue factors (PAI-1, selectins) produced by injured endothelium which initiates the coagulation cascade; and reduced production of natural antithrombotics (t-PA, PGI_2) at the site of vascular injury due to the endothelial cell damage [25]. Moreover, small vein endothelium appears to be more susceptible to traumatic endothelial damage, leading to a more consistent production of prothrombotic factors. The presence of the catheter itself may provide a thrombogenic surface.

The early formation (within 24 h) of a "fibrin sleeve" after the placement of a vascular catheter has been observed since the mid-1960s; in most cases, the portion of the catheter closer to the introduction point was mainly involved [26]. A study published in 1998 [27] was performed by controlling venous catheters inserted into the anterior caval vein of rats at scheduled intervals. It reported that the formation of the "fibrin sleeve" was an almost constant phenomenon when a foreign body was introduced into the blood stream. Normally it began to form at the point where the endothelium was damaged. The fibrin sleeve was observed in most cases at the insertion point and less frequently on the catheter tip; as previously reported, it was already detectable after the first 24 h and only in a minority of cases gave rise to an organized thrombosis.

It is also important to consider the hypercoagulability linked to the presence of cancer, particularly evident for hematological malignancies [28]. Most of the patients requiring long-term venous access are oncologic patients; this is a major and peculiar risk for developing CRDVT. International practice guidelines for treatment and prophylaxis of catheter-related DVT specifically for cancer patients have been recently published [29].

10.2   Diagnosis

PICC-related deep vein thrombosis can present a large spectrum of symptoms, ranging from total absence of symptoms to a superior vena cava syndrome or pulmonary embolism.

At one end of the spectrum, PRDVT may be entirely asymptomatic. In a number of observational studies [22, 30, 34], asymptomatic thrombosis represents up to 95 % of all the PRDVT.

For what concerns symptomatic PICC-related thrombosis, the most common reported symptoms in literature are variously combined:

- Upper arm swelling (40–50 % of all symptomatic thrombosis)
- Sense of heaviness (30–40 %)
- Pain (35–40 %)
- Skin temperature increase (15–20 %)
- Forearm swelling (15 %)
- Limb cyanosis (5–10 %)
- Dilation of subcutaneous veins (4–5 %)
- Jugular vein distension (2–3 %)

Although episodic reports, a recent meta-analysis comparing PICC- and CVC-related DVT reported no pulmonary embolism in comparative studies [4]. Anyway, the paucity of studies available at this time does not allow us to ignore signs and symptoms of pulmonary embolism (cough, dyspnea, thoracic pain, palpitations) as a suspicion for the presence of PICC-related deep vein thrombosis.

Compressive ultrasound examination (CUE), which has proven to have in adults high specificity (86–100 %), sensitivity (78–100 %), and negative predictive value

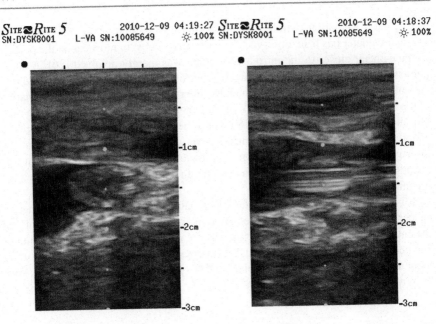

Figs. 10.1 and 10.2 Echographic image of a PICC surrounded by thrombus in axillary vein, transverse and longitudinal section

in diagnosis of deep venous thrombosis [31–33], with a quasi-ubiquitary availability and a total absence of invasivity, turns out to be the ideal tool for the screening of PICC-related venous thrombosis [34].

The most recent guidelines of the American College of Chest Physicians [41] suggest (Grade 2C) an initial evaluation with combined modality US (compression with either Doppler or color Doppler) over other initial tests in patients suspected of having upper extremity deep vein thrombosis; only if initial US examination is negative, in the presence of high risk or high clinical suspicion, further testing with serial US, CT scan, or MRI (Grade 2C) was suggested.

In case of suspicion for the presence of PRDVT, a complete examination of the upper limb and neck vessels by means of a duplex ultrasound and Doppler or color Doppler has to be performed. At the same time, the whole arm and the exit site must be inspected to exclude infections, known to be an additional risk for DVT in the underlying vessel and a possible complication in case of infected thrombus [10]. Diagnostic criteria for DVT include incompressibility of the vein and, in most cases, direct visualization of PICC-surrounding thrombus [35] (Figs. 10.1 and 10.2)

This test is considered diagnostic if positive and does not need further evaluation with more invasive diagnostic tools, according to the above cited ACCP guidelines and to less recent but still valid guidelines and reviews [42, 43]. Initial evaluation in case of clinical suspicion or high-risk patients must be available in any PICC team with echographic-trained personnel.

10.3   Therapy

For what concerns the treatment of a PICC-related deep vein thrombosis, we refer to the above cited ACCP guidelines (*Chest* 2012), to the international guidelines for CVC-related thrombosis in patients with cancer [29], and to the review "Management of occlusion and thrombosis associated with long-term indwelling central venous catheters" (Baskin, *Lancet* 2009).

In particular:

- The catheter must not be removed if functional and needed and if its tip is correctly positioned.
- Early removal of the catheter is necessary only in case of pulmonary embolism or infected thrombophlebitis.
- In any other case, removal of the catheter must be preceded by 3–5 days of effective anticoagulation (Figs. 10.3, 10.4, 10.5, 10.6, 10.7 and 10.8).
- Acute anticoagulation must be performed with full-dose LMWH or fondaparinux.
- Long-term full-dose anticoagulation in oncologic patients is mandatory with LMWH or fondaparinux; for non-oncologic patients, VKAs can be considered.
- Anticoagulation must be continued as long as the catheter is maintained.
- The duration of anticoagulation after catheter withdrawal is still debated.

The grades of evidence for the advised therapies reported in ACCP guidelines 2012 are:

- For the treatment of superficial vein thrombosis (basilic vein is considered by some authors as a "large vein," not a "deep vein"): prophylactic dose of fondaparinux or LMWH for 45 days (Grade 2B)
- For the acute anticoagulation for upper arm deep vein thrombosis (UEDVT): parenteral anticoagulation with UEDVT or fondaparinux (Grade 1b)
- For the long-term anticoagulation for UEDVT: if CVC-related, not to remove catheter if functional and needed (Grade 2C); anticoagulation as long as the catheter is maintained in situ (Grade 1C for oncologic patients, Grade 2C for other patients); minimum duration of anticoagulation of 3 months if catheter is removed (Grade 2B)

10.4   Prevention

Efforts to use pharmacologic prophylaxis with heparin, ASA, or warfarin to reduce catheter-related DVT have not resulted in any consistent conclusion [36, 37]. In particular, a 2008 huge meta-analysis about thromboprophylaxis for patients with cancer and central venous catheters reports that the balance of benefits and downsides of thromboprophylaxis in cancer patients with CVC remains uncertain [38]. More recently ACCP guidelines 2012, dealing with patients with cancer and indwelling central venous catheters, suggest evidence against routine prophylaxis with LMWH or LDUH (Grade B) and VKAs (Grade 2C); on the contrary, for patients with additional thrombosis risk factors, a prophylactic dose of LMWH or LDUH is suggested (Grade 2B).

Other studies aimed to reduce complications of central venous catheterization led to the development of techniques, such as real-time ultrasound guidance, that minimizing the traumatism on endothelium in fact reduced the risk of developing catheter-related thrombosis [39].

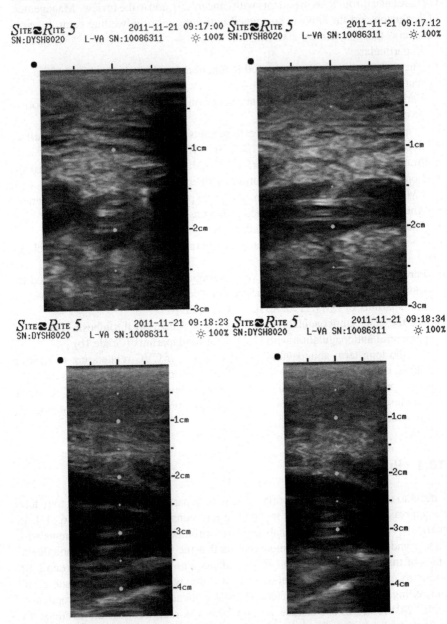

Figs. 10.3, 10.4, 10.5, 10.6, 10.7 and 10.8 Echographic image of a PICC surrounded by thrombus in brachial vein, extended in axillary and subclavian till the confluence with internal jugular vein

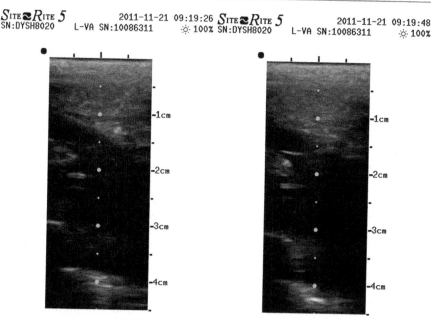

Figs. 10.3, 10.4, 10.5, 10.6, 10.7 and 10.8   (continued)

With the widespread diffusion of new positioning techniques, the evolution of materials and technology of devices, and the development of new intravenous onco-logic therapies, the diffusion of central venous access in the last 20 years has importantly grown; for this reason, medium- and long-term complications are more and more observed, and a lot of effort has been made in finding a way to prevent them.

Many reviews and meta-analysis have been published on risk factors, prevention, and treatment of CVC-related thrombosis [4, 6, 9, 29, 44]; the huge heterogenicity of studies design and inclusion criteria led to scarcely important indications, as the identification of risk factors turned out to be very different from study to study.

In 2007 the Italian consensus group for central venous access (GAVeCeLT) published on JAVA a paper concerning the catheter-related central venous thrombosis ("the development of a nationwide consensus paper in Italy") [40], more recently focused on PICC-related complications, that can be referred to as a "bundle" for prevention.

As regards prevention, according to ACCP 2012 guidelines, SOR 2008 guidelines, international 2012 guidelines for CRDVT in cancer patients, and GAVeCeLT consensus, we suggest the following points:

- Echographic complete evaluation of all upper limb and neck veins, in order to identify the bigger and straighter vein to be cannulated.
- Preferential right side approach.
- Avoiding paretic arm when possible.
- The smallest needed catheter in the biggest vein.
- Real-time ultrasound guidance.

- Aseptic technique of positioning and maximal barrier protection.
- Correct localization of catheter tip in proximity of atriocaval junction, when possible with ECG intracavitary technique.
- Catheter stabilization with sutureless devices.
- Careful maintenance of the catheter for preventing infections.
- For patients with additional risk factors (previous DVT, sepsis, cancer + another DVT risk factor), a prophylactic dose of LMWH or LDUH can be considered.

References

1. Kalso E (1985) A short history of central venous catheterization. Acta Anaesthesiol Scand 81:7–10
2. Smith JR, Friedell ML, Cheatham ML et al (1998) Peripherally inserted central catheters revisited. Am J Surg 176:208–211
3. Souza FF, Otero HJ, Erturk M et al (2009) Venous thrombosis in an outpatient oncologic center: distribution, type, and comorbidities. Ultrasound Q 25:145–150
4. Chopra V, Anand S, Hickner A, Buist M, Rogers MAM, Saint S, Flanders SA (2013) Risk of venous thromboembolism associated with peripherally inserted central catheters: a systematic review and meta-analysis. Lancet 382:311–325
5. Pikwer A, Akeson J, Lindgren S (2004) Complications associated with peripheral or central routes for central venous cannulation. Anaesthesia 67:65–71
6. Verso M, Agnelli G (2003) Venous thromboembolism associated with long-term use of central venous catheters in cancer patients. J Clin Oncol 21(19):3665–3675
7. Acedo Sanchez JD et al (2007) Catheter-related thrombosis: a critical review. Support Cancer Ther 4(3):145–151
8. Geerts WH, Heit JA, Clagett GP et al (2001) Prevention of venous thromboembolism. Chest 119(1):132–175
9. Kuter DJ (2004) Thrombotic complications of central venous catheters in cancer patients. Oncologist 9:207–216
10. Boersma RS, Jie KS, Verbon A et al (2008) Thrombotic and infectious complications of central venous catheters in patients with hematological malignancies. Ann Oncol 19:433–442
11. Biffi R, De Braud F, Orsi F et al (1998) Totally implantable central venous access ports for long-term chemotherapy. A prospective study analyzing complications and costs in 333 devices with a minimum 180 days of follow-up. Ann Oncol 9:767–773
12. Timsit JF, Farkas JC, Boyer JM et al (1998) Central vein catheter-related thrombosis in intensive care patients: incidence, risk factors, and relationship with catheter-related sepsis. Chest 114:207–213
13. Merrer J, De Jonghe B, Golliot F et al; French Catheter Study Group in Intensive Care (2001) Complications of femoral and subclavian venous catheterization in critically-ill patients: a randomized controlled trial. JAMA 286:700–707
14. Monreal M, Lafoz E, Ruiz J, Valls R, Alastrue A (1991) Upper-extremity deep venous thrombosis and pulmonary embolism. A prospective study. Chest 99:280–283
15. Monreal M, Raventos A, Lerma R et al (1994) Pulmonary embolism in patients with upper extremity DVT associated to venous central lines – a prospective study. Thromb Haemost 72:548–550
16. Pradoni P, Polistene P, Bernardi E et al (1997) Upper-extremity deep vein thrombosis: risk factors, diagnosis, and complications. Arch Intern Med 157:57–62
17. Paauw JD, Borders H, Ingalls N et al (2008) The incidence of PICC line-associated thrombosis with and without the use of prophylactic anticoagulants. J Parenter Enteral Nutr 32:443–447
18. Chemaly R, Barbara de Parres J, Rehm S et al (2002) Venous thrombosis associated with peripherally inserted central catheters: a retrospective analysis of the Cleveland Clinic experience. Clin Infect Dis 34:1179–1183

19. Grove JR, Pevec WC (2000) Venous thrombosis related to peripherally inserted central catheters. J Vasc Interv Radiol 11:837–840

20. Liem TK, Yanit KE et al (2010) Peripherally inserted central catheter usage patterns and associated symptomatic upper extremity venous thrombosis. J Vasc Surg 55:761–767

21. Abdullah BJ, Mohammad N (2005) Incidence of upper limb venous thrombosis associated with peripherally inserted central catheters (PICC). Br J Radiol 78:596–600

22. Trerotola SO, Stavropoulos SW et al (2010) Triple-lumen peripherally inserted central catheter in patients in the critical care unit: prospective evaluation. Radiology 256:312–320

23. Baskin JL, Pui C-H et al (2009) Management of occlusion and thrombosis associated with long-term indwelling central venous catheters. Lancet 374:159–169

24. Nifong TP, McDevitt TJ (2011) The effect of catheter to vein ratio on blood flow rates in a simulated model of peripherally inserted central venous catheters. Chest 140(1):48–53

25. Armstrong AW, Golan DE, Tashjian AH, Armstrong E (2008) Principles of pharmacology: the pathophysiologic basis of drug therapy. Wolters Kluwer Health/Lippincott Williams & Wilkins, Philadelphia, p 396

26. Hoshal VL, Ause RG et al (1971) Fibrin sleeve formation on indwelling subclavian central venous catheter. Arch Surg 102:235–258

27. Xiang DZ, Verbeken MD et al (1998) Composition and formation of the sleeve enveloping a central venous catheter. J Vasc Surg 28:260–271

28. Boersma RS, Schouten HC (2010) Clinical practices concerning central venous catheters in haematological patients. Eur J Oncol Nurs 14:200–204

29. Debourdeau P, Farge D, Beckers M et al (2013) International clinical practice guidelines for the treatment and prophylaxis of thrombosis associated with central venous catheters in patients with cancer. J Thromb Haemost 11:71–80

30. Yi XL, Chen J, Li J, Feng L, Wang Y, Zhu JA, Shen E, Hu B (2014) Risk factors associated with PICC-related upper extremity venous thrombosis in cancer patients. J Clin Nurs 23(5–6):837–843. doi:10.1111/jocn.12227

31. Mustafa BO, Rathbun SW, Whitsett TL, Raskob GE (2002) Sensitivity and specificity of ultrasonography in the diagnosis of upper extremity deep vein thrombosis: a systematic review. Arch Intern Med 162:401–404

32. Sajid MS, Ahmed N, Desai M, Baker D, Hamilton G (2007) Upper limb deep vein thrombosis: a literature review to streamline the protocol for management. Acta Haematol 118:10–18

33. Baarslag HJ, van Beek EJ, Koopman MM, Reekers JA (2002) Prospective study of color duplex ultrasonography compared with contrast venography in patients suspected of having deep venous thrombosis of the upper extremities. Ann Intern Med 136:865–872

34. Bonizzoli M, Batacchi S, Cianchi G et al (2011) Peripherally inserted central venous catheters and central venous catheters related thrombosis in post-critical patients. Intensive Care Med 37(2):284–289

35. Zierler BK (2004) Ultrasonography and diagnosis of venous thromboembolism. Circulation 109:I-9–I-14

36. Verso M, Agnelli G, Bertoglio S et al (2005) Enoxaparin for the prevention of venous thromboembolism associated with central vein catheter: a double-blind, placebo-controlled, randomized study in cancer patients. J Clin Oncol 23:4057–4062

37. Massicotte P, Julian JA, Gent M et al (2003) An open-label randomized controlled trial of low molecular weight heparin for the prevention of central venous line-related thrombotic complications in children: the PROTEKT trial. Thromb Res 109:101–108

38. Akl EA, Kamath G, Yosuico V et al (2008) Thromboprophylaxis for patients with cancer and central venous catheters: a systematic review and a meta-analysis. Cancer 112(11):2483–2492

39. Mc Gee DC, Gould K (2003) Preventing complications of central venous catheterization. N Engl J Med 348:1123–1133

40. Campisi C, Biffi R, Pittiruti M (2007) Catheter-related central venous thrombosis: the development of a nationwide consensus paper in Italy. JAVA 12:38–46

41. Guyatt GH, Akl EA, Crowther M et al (2012) Antithrombotic therapy and prevention of thrombosis, 9th ed: American College of Chest Physicians Evidence-Based Clinical Practice Guidelines. Chest 141:7S–47S

42. Zierler BK (2004) Ultrasonography and diagnosis of venous thromboembolism. Circulation 109:I-9-I-14
43. Kearon C, Ginsberg JS, Hirsh J (1998) The role of venous ultrasonography in the diagnosis of suspected deep venous thrombosis and pulmonary embolism. Ann Intern Med 129(12):1044–9
44. Debourdeau P, Kassab Chahmi D, Le Gal G et al (2009) 2008 SOR guidelines for the prevention and treatment of thrombosis associated with central venous catheters in patients with cancer: report from the working group. Annals of Oncology 20:1459–1471

Maneuvers, Precautions, and Tricks for PICC Positioning Procedure

Antonius J.H. van Boxtel

11.1 Introduction

Since the first publication by Hoshal [1] on the use of peripherally inserted catheters (PICCs), there have been changes in catheter materials, insertion techniques, securement and care, and maintenance.

Based on the consensus paper by Moureau et al. [2], all central venous access devices should be inserted using ultrasound for vein detection and vein access. For that reason, this chapter will focus on useful suggestions to help you in finding the right vein and getting access to the vein using ultrasound and Modified Seldinger Technique (MST). In the process of insertion and care and maintenance of PICC, challenges and difficulties reduce the success rate of PICC use. This chapter offers well-known and unknown tips to prevent and to treat complications during insertion of a PICC.

11.2 Preparation

Correct and honest information to the patient is an important part of preparation for PICC insertion and will help the patient to better understand and be more relaxed. If the patient is stressed and scared for the procedure, a formulation of premedication or sedation for the patient can help to have a successful and less stressful PICC insertion.

The inserter should be able to have an upright or, if preferred, sitting position. The patient on a comfortable bed or stretcher offers the best circumstances for a relaxed and least demanding procedure. A spacious room and enough light that is not blinding your ultrasound screen are basic conditions to improve your outcome on PICC insertion.

Depending on the location for PICC insertion, bedside or under fluoroscopy has an influence on techniques that can be used.

A.J.H. van Boxtel, RN, MSc, VA-BC
Department of Vascular Access, Infusion Innovations, Nimrodlaan 12,
Bilthoven 3721BX, The Netherlands
e-mail: ton@infu-in.com

S. Sandrucci, B. Mussa (eds.), *Peripherally Inserted Central Venous Catheters*,
DOI 10.1007/978-88-470-5665-7_11, © Springer-Verlag Italia 2014

11.3   PICC Insertion Using Fluoroscopy

Fluoroscopy is an imaging technique that uses X-ray to obtain real-time moving images of the internal structures of a patient through the use of a fluoroscope. In its simplest form, a fluoroscope consists of an X-ray source and fluorescent screen between which a patient is placed. Modern fluoroscopes couple the screen to an X-ray image intensifier and a video camera allowing the images to be recorded and played on a monitor [3]. Under fluoroscopy, a long guidewire is used for PICC insertion. After vein access, the guidewire is positioned at the desired depth for tip positioning. The PICC can be trimmed in the correct length based on the total length of the guidewire minus the remaining external length. After inserting the sheath dilator and removing the dilator, the PICC can be advanced over the guidewire into the correct position. Therefore, a stylet or stiffener is not needed. The wire will be removed and the procedure can be completed.

Fluoroscopy is also used if the bedside procedure shows resistance that cannot be solved and all the bedside tricks do not have the optimal result. The image can show different malpositions. The tip can be up in the jugular vein or can go across into the opposite brachiocephalic or innominate vein.

If tricks like different positions of the head and arm do not allow tip placement in the SVC, a "steering" guidewire with an adjustable tip can be used to enter the superior vena cava and to guide the PICC over this wire into the correct position.

11.4   Bedside PICC Insertion

Most PICCs can be successfully inserted at the bedside. A dedicated team of experts have a success rate up to 98 %. Complicating factors are previous venous access, vein damage, thromboses, and infections that can cause obstruction and formation of collaterals.

Thorough anamneses of the patient history and the trajectory of the PICC can help you to choose the best site and prevent unnecessary needlesticks and tissue damage. Depending on the patient's history with venous access and or thrombosis, this might include a duplex ultrasound.

Duplex ultrasound combines Doppler flow information and conventional imaging information. It shows how blood is flowing through veins and measures the speed of flow of blood. It can also be useful to estimate the diameter of a vein and possible obstruction of the vein.

11.5   Vein

To distinguish the vein from the artery, controlled compression of the vein and artery will show pulsation if the artery is partly compressed. The vein can be compressed completely, while the artery has a higher counterpressure. Compression of the vein also gives you information on the condition of the vein. If compression of

Fig. 11.1 Vein – Catheter
ratio

Minimum size of vein needed

PICC diameter in French

Vein diameter in mm   4   5   6

Fig. 11.2 T-probe with
double image

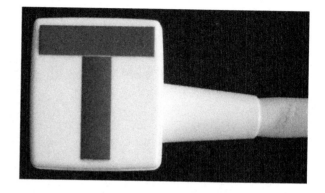

the vein is not or only partly possible, this might be an indication of a thrombosis in this area of the vein. The use of Doppler, if available, can help to determine the flow and possible obstruction.

The size of the vein is an important predictor of minimal blood flow that is needed to prevent thrombosis related to stasis.

The easiest way to determine and remember the minimal diameter of the vein is to use the number of the catheter French size and to take that number in millimeters. For example, for a 4 French PICC, you need a minimal diameter of 4 mm; 5 French, 5 mm diameter; etc. (Fig. 11.1).

The diameter of the vein should be measured without tourniquet.

If the desired diameter cannot be found in the ideal zone for upper arm needle insertion with ultrasound guidance [4] on the upper arm, you can choose for tunneling to a more appropriate exit site.

11.6   Vein Access

For getting access to the desired vein, you can use two types of probes or transducer.

A linear probe can be used for PICC insertion or a T-probe (Fig. 11.2).

The most frequent used probe is the linear probe that allows you switch between in-plane (Fig. 11.3) and out-of-plane approach (Fig. 11.4). Both options are used by clinicians. Personal preference is mainly based on training. The T-probe (Fig. 11.4) gives you two images at the same time without the need to turn the probe during vein access and has an in- and out-of-plane image on the screen.

Fig. 11.3 In plane
(with permission
of Dr Rafiq Mikhael)

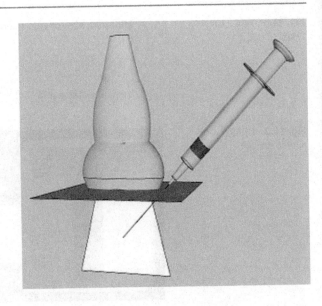

Fig. 11.4 Out of plane (with
permission of Dr Rafiq
Mikhael)

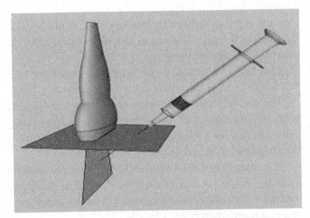

Particularly during the initial training period, a needle guide can help to position the needle very precisely in the beam and have better visualization of vein entry. Most clinicians do not use a needle guide anymore after they have sufficient control of the ultrasound and the complete procedure. The angle of the needle should be lowered to allow the guidewire to enter the vein more easily even in a small vein. The bevel or opening of the needle should always point forward.

The use of a tourniquet creates counterpressure and increases resistance in the vein preventing the needlepoint from compressing the vein before penetrating the vein wall. Increased vein pressure enlarges the diameter at the time of vein puncture resulting in a higher success rate for vein access.

Ultrasound should be used at all times during vein access and can also confirm the guidewire being in the vein.

11.7   PICC Advancing

Depending on the size of the PICC, the flexibility of the catheter, and the condition of the veins, the risk of obstruction during advancement of the PICC is real. To be in control of the situation and to allow the PICC to go with the blood flow, advancing the catheter should be done slowly. When the tip of the PICC is in the axillary vein, the patient should move the ear towards the shoulder of the side of insertion. By bending the jugular vein away, the tip should go towards the SVC. In most cases of bedside PICC procedures, a PICC can be supported with a stylet or stiffener in the catheter to prevent easy kinking or looping of the PICC. The stiffener can be advanced till 1 cm before the distal opening. The stiffener has a sharp point and can cause vein rupture if pointing out of the tip of the PICC. If a double- or triple-lumen PICC is still coiling despite of the stiffener, the guidewire can be introduced in the other lumen to have an even stiffer catheter. Of course the guidewire should have at least 1 cm on the outside on the proximal end to be able to remove the wire after tip positioning.

Together with lifting and/or moving the arm upwards, it might allow the catheter tip to pass more easily and increase successful tip positioning of the PICC.

A power flush with normal saline during catheter advancement might give some stiffness and increase outcome on tip positioning.

At all times, prevent the catheter from touching the skin and prevent the catheter from coming in contact with the gloves. Contact with the skin can be prevented by placing a sterile gauze between the skin and catheter. For advancing the catheter, a sterile forceps can be used.

A simple technique to know if the tip is in the jugular vein is to do a power flush with normal saline. This can only be performed if the patient is awake and able to respond. Instruct the patient to concentrate on the neck at the insertion side and to let you know if anything is felt after the power flush. If not, you have a clear indication that the tip is not in the jugular vein. An alternative is to place the ultrasound probe low in the neck of the insertion side at the jugular vein. An expert is able to see if the catheter is in the jugular vein.

After advancing the PICC for the desired length, confirmation of the tip position is needed. X-ray confirmation is still used but is often replaced with ECG P-wave confirmation depending on the availability of ECG for tip confirmation. The ECG method has clear advantages in terms of accuracy, cost-effectiveness, and feasibility in conditions where X-ray control may be difficult or expensive to obtain. The method is quite simple, easy to learn and to teach, noninvasive, easy to reproduce, safe, and apt to minimize malpositions due to failure of entering the SVC [5]. PICC insertion does not have a risk for pneumothorax, and an X-ray is not needed to exclude this risk.

11.8 Repositioning of PICC

Two types of malpositioning can occur:
- Malpositioning during the insertion procedure
  - This situation allows to pull the catheter as far as the tip being in the axillary vein and advance the PICC using the described tips.
- Malpositioning after finishing the procedure
  - This is a procedure with a higher risk for contamination. This can only be done if the inserter is able to go back to a sterile environment and the PICC is not touched or touching the skin during the repositioning procedure. If the initial procedure was already complicated, the best option is to ask the interventional radiologist to assist using imaging and advanced techniques with contrast and steering guidewires.

11.9 Renewal of a PICC

For the renewal of a PICC, we can also have two options:
- Renewal at another site, normally the opposite side of the patient
  - If the situation allows to remove the existing PICC before inserting a new PICC, that is preferred. In case of a suspected PICC infection, the best option is to remove the PICC and wait 24 h before inserting a new PICC.
- Renewal of the PICC using the same insertion site
  - This option is only available if the insertion site is not suspected for infection. Indications are as follows:
    - Need for a multi-lumen PICC
    - A ruptured or broken PICC
    - If the PICC is partly removed but still in the vein

Prepare the skin and PICC using skin antisepsis and go back to a sterile environment. The outer part of the PICC is wrapped in gauze and if needed pulled back till only 15 cm is in situ. Cut the catheter and insert the guidewire in the remaining part. Remove the old PICC completely leaving the guidewire inside. Change gloves and proceed placing the new PICC.

References

1. Hoshal VL (1975) Total intravenous nutrition with peripherally inserted silicone elastomer central venous catheters. Arch Surg 110(5):644–646
2. Moureau N, Lamperti M, Kelly LJ, Dawson R, Elbarbary M, van Boxtel AJH, Pittiruti M (2013) Evidence-based consensus on the insertion of central venous access devices: definition of minimal requirements for training, Br J Anaesth 110(3):1–10
3. Wikipedia. http://en.wikipedia.org/wiki/Fluoroscopy
4. Dawson RB (2011) PICC Zone Insertion Method™ : a systematic approach to determine the ideal insertion site for PICCs in the upper arm. JAVA 16(3):P156–P165
5. Pittiruti M, Scoppettuolo G, La Greca A, Emoli A, Brutti A, Ivano M, Dolcetti L, Taraschi C, de Pascale G (2008) The EKG method for positioning the tip of PICCs: results from two preliminary studies. JAVA 13(4):179–186

The "Off-Label" Use of PICCs

12

Mauro Pittiruti

12.1 Introduction

When dealing with the topic "The Off-Label Use of PICCs," an appropriate definition of our terminology is mandatory.

What are we talking about when we talk about "PICCs" ? PICC is notoriously the acronym for "peripherally inserted central catheters," though the device known and used as "PICC" in the world of vascular access today is not just simply a central catheter which is inserted through a peripheral vein. Many other peripherally inserted central catheters have been used in the past or are currently used in selected patients, though it is hard to consider them as analogues to the device that we currently define as "PICC."

In the last decades of the twentieth century, several central catheters have been marketed and clinically used for peripheral insertion, such as drum cartridge (Abbott) or CavaFix (Bbraun). These ancestors of the current PICCs were made of materials far less biocompatible than today (polyethylene, first-generation polyurethanes), and they were inserted with an obsolete methodology (direct insertion of the catheter in a palpable or visible vein of the antecubital fossa by the "catheter through the needle" technique). Later on, in the 1990s, new peripherally inserted central venous devices – made of more biocompatible materials (silicone or third-generation polyurethane) – were introduced in the clinical arena, but still the methodology of insertion consisted in the "blind" cannulation of an antecubital vein. Only in the first years of the twenty-first century, a "new" device was designed, which was still named "PICC," but it was obviously a different vascular access device, due to the innovative methodology of insertion (ultrasound-guided cannulation of the deep veins of the arm, by the modified Seldinger technique); a new term

M. Pittiruti, MD
Department of Surgery, Catholic University Hospital, Rome, Italy

Dip. Scienze Chirurgiche, Università Cattolica del Sacro Cuore,
largo Francesco Vito 1, 00168 Rome, Italy
e-mail: mauro.pittiruti@rm.unicatt.it

S. Sandrucci, B. Mussa (eds.), *Peripherally Inserted Central Venous Catheters*,
DOI 10.1007/978-88-470-5665-7_12, © Springer-Verlag Italia 2014

like "ultrasound-PICC," "US-PICC," or "echo-PICC" would have been more appropriate to mark the difference from its predecessors.

In a every selected population of patients, i.e., neonates, some central catheters are threaded via a superficial peripheral vein, and they are sometimes defined as "PICCs." Nonetheless, these devices – which should more appropriately be defined as "epicutaneo-caval catheters" (ECCs) – are completely different from ultrasound-guided PICCs [1]. As a matter of fact, ECCs have a clinical role exclusively in neonates or small infants; they are inserted in superficial veins of the limbs or of the scalp that are directly visible through the skin or visualized by near-infrared devices [2]; their caliber ranges between 1Fr and 2.7Fr, so that they are inappropriate for hemodynamic monitoring and blood sampling; the position of their tip is often "almost central" (anywhere in the superior or inferior vena cava). On the contrary, the devices that we currently define as "PICCs" cannot be inserted in neonates and small infants (which rarely have veins at the arm with a caliber > 3 mm); they are inserted in deep veins of the arm visualized and cannulated by ultrasound guidance; their caliber is 3Fr or more, so that they can be used for hemodynamic monitoring and blood sampling; the position of the tip is meant to be appropriately "central," i.e., in the proximity of the cavo-atrial junction.

So, when we are talking about "PICCs" today, we should properly refer to central catheters of silicone or third-generation polyurethane or power-injectable polyurethane, with caliber ranging from 3Fr to 6Fr; single, double, or triple lumen; and inserted by the modified Seldinger technique and ultrasound guidance in the deep veins of the arm (basilic vein, brachial veins, or – in obese patients – cephalic vein), with the tip ideally located at the cavo-atrial junction [3].

Such methodology of insertion is currently described and recommended in the vast majority of IFU (instructions for use) from different manufacturers, and it should be regarded as the "in-label," officially approved methodology of insertion.

On the other hand, as regards the indications for clinical use, most manufacturers recommend that the PICCs should be used for any kind of intravenous infusion (including infusion of vesicant drugs, parenteral nutrition, blood or blood products) as well as for blood sampling and hemodynamic monitoring (which basically includes the estimate of central venous pressure and the measurement of the oxygen saturation in mixed venous blood).

Therefore, when we talk about the "off-label" use of PICCs, we should address at least three different aspects:
- Atypical or "off-label" techniques of insertion
- Atypical or "off-label" sites of insertion
- Atypical or "off-label" indications for use

12.2 Atypical or "Off-Label" Technique of Insertion

The technique of PICC insertion as described by the IFU usually consists in the ultrasound-guided puncture and cannulation of a deep vein of the arm located in the area proximal to the antecubital fossa and distal to the axilla, typically the basilic vein or one of the brachial veins [3]. These are considered as "deep" veins. In obese patients, another possible option is the cephalic vein at the arm, which usually is a very superficial vein (less than 5 mm from the skin surface), but it may become quite deep – and thus more stable and more appropriate for PICC placement – when the subcutaneous fat is increased.

The cannulation of the vein is achieved by the so-called modified Seldinger technique (which means puncture by needle, insertion of a guidewire through the needle, removal of the needle, insertion of a micro-introducer-dilator over the guidewire, removal of the wire and of the dilator, insertion of the catheter through the introducer, peel away removal of the micro-introducer). At the end of the maneuver, as described by the IFU, the site of venipuncture corresponds with the exit site.

Sometimes, it may be clinically needed that the exit site should be distant from the puncture site and this can be achieved by tunneling the catheter for a short tract. Tunnelization of PICCs, though it is considered an "off-label" variation of the insertion technique, is of great interest, and it is extremely useful in several clinical situations [4].

The ideal exit site for PICCs is usually considered the middle third of the upper arm (considering as "upper arm" the tract of the limb between the axilla and the antecubital fossa). With reference to the Zone Insertion Method recently described by Rob Dawson [5], this "ideal" area for the exit site would correspond to the "green" zone. Sometimes the veins of the patient may be too small in the "green" zone for the safe placement of the desired catheter. The universal recommendation in this regard is that the vein should have an inner diameter at least three times larger than the external diameter of the catheter. This implies that a 3Fr catheter would ask for a 3 mm vein (or larger), a 4Fr catheter for a 4 mm vein (or larger), and so on. If the veins in the "green" area are too small for the desired catheter size, we have only two options: either we choose a smaller catheter size or we look for a larger vein, more proximally, in Dawson's "yellow" area. In the latter situation, tunneling the catheter for a small tract (3–6 cm) may allow us to achieve an appropriate location of the puncture site (i.e., an appropriate vein size) in the "yellow" area and simultaneously an appropriate location of the exit site in the "green" area (Fig. 12.1).

Tunneling is a very simple procedure which can be performed with any PICC (of any material, of any company), using either a small needle cannula or a dedicated tunneler.

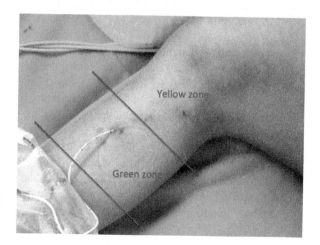

Fig. 12.1 Tunneled PICC: puncture site in the "yellow" zone, exit site in the "green" zone

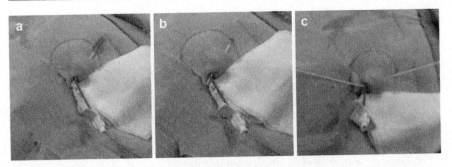

Fig. 12.2 Tunneling via a 14G needle cannula (description in the text)

Fig. 12.3 Glue is used to
seal both the puncture site
and the exit site

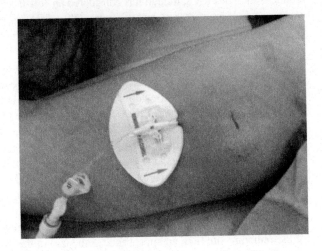

The needle cannula technique (Fig. 12.2) requires either a 16G cannula (for 3Fr PICCs) or a 14G cannula (for 4–5Fr PICCs). The same inexpensive 52 mm needle cannulas used for common peripheral i.v. lines are used. Soon after the insertion of the guidewire and/or of the micro-introducer-dilator into the vein, the incision on the skin is slightly enlarged by a #11 scalpel; after local subcutaneous anesthesia (few ml of ropivacaine or mepivacaine), the needle cannula is inserted in the skin few cm below the puncture site, exactly where the exit site has been planned (Fig. 12.2a); the needle is removed, the cone of the cannula is trimmed (Fig. 12.2b), and the catheter is threaded into the cannula (Fig. 12.2c). After the cannula is removed, the catheter is threaded into the micro-introducer (so called "anterograde" tunnelization). Both the exit site and the incision at the puncture site are sealed with cyanoacrylate glue (Fig. 12.3).

Another possible option is the use of a dedicated PICC tunneler, available through different companies (Cook Medical, for instance). This is a metallic, non-sharp tunneler 12–15 cm long, which is inserted in the subcutaneous tissue through a small skin incision, several cm distally to the puncture site. Even in this case, it would be an "anterograde" tunnelization.

The anterograde tunneling maneuver can be done with any PICC, and it is the only option for PICCs which must be trimmed distally (i.e., the vast majority of PICCs commercially available). When dealing with PICCs which must be trimmed proximally (such as "Groshong PICC," Bard, or "PICC Easy," Vygon), the tunnelization is obviously retrograde and somehow easier.

Tunneling is particularly useful in pediatric patients, where veins are usually of reduced size and PICC placement is possible only by choosing veins very close to the axilla.

In summary, tunneling allows a "high" puncture of the deep veins of the arm, with several advantages:

- It increases the indications of PICCs.
- It allows PICC use in situations where tunneled catheters are explicitly recommended by national guidelines or by hospital policies (such as in the UK, where the guidelines of the British Committee for Standards in Haematology recommend that in bone marrow transplant, patients only tunneled catheters should be used).
- It reduces the risk of catheter-related bloodstream infection (since it reduces the extraluminal contamination of the catheter).
- It reduces the risk of thrombosis (since it allows to cannulate larger veins).
- Also, if a cuffed PICC is used (such as Pro-Line, Medcomp), the PICC becomes a long-term venous access device, since the coupling of tunnel + cuff protects from extraluminal contamination and increases the stability of the catheter, making it less prone to dislocation.

Tunneling of PICCs has been extensively used in recent years by our PICC team (Catholic University Hospital, Rome, Italy) and by several clinical groups all over the world (Gail Egan and coworkers, USA; Michele Di Giacomo and coworkers, UK; Gloria Ortiz Miluy and coworkers, Spain), with very good clinical outcomes:

- It is technically easy and safe for the patient.
- Patient compliance is very good.
- With a proper technique of tunnelization (i.e., expansion of the subcutaneous tissue by local anesthetic or by saline infusion; use of blunt tunneler), the occurrence of hematomas is very unusual, even in patients with coagulation disorders.
- Tunneling does not conflict with the adoption of the method of intracavitary ECG for tip location, though when using a cuffed catheter, pre-insertion landmark-based estimate of the length of the catheter should be particularly accurate, so as to achieve simultaneously a correct placement of the tip at the cavo-atrial junction and a correct position of the cuff inside the tunnel, at no less than 2 cm from the exit site, as recommended by the current guidelines.

Tunneling is of great value also for PICCs inserted in atypical or "off-label" veins, as it will be discussed in the next paragraphs.

12.3   Atypical or "Off-Label" Site of Insertion

Though the IFU of most commercially available PICCs usually take into consideration only the cannulation of the basilic vein, the brachial veins, or the cephalic vein, PICCs can be inserted with relevant clinical advantages in many other veins which can be punctured and cannulated by ultrasound guidance.

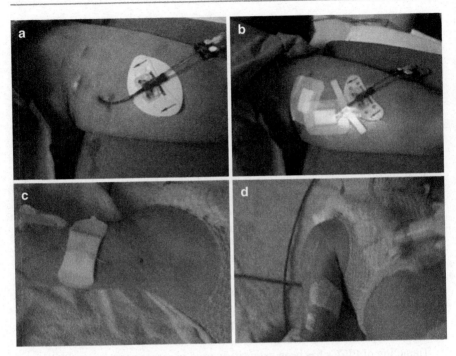

Fig. 12.4 Tunneled PICC in an adult (**a**, **b**) and in a pediatric patient (**c**, **d**)

12.3.1 Axillary Vein at the Upper Arm or at the Axilla

In some cases, as described above, basilic and brachial veins may be unavailable for PICC insertion (either because too small or occluded by thrombosis). This typically happens in infants and children or in skinny, malnourished aged patients or in patients with history of multiple PICC placements. In such cases, the axillary vein can be safely punctured and cannulated in its extrathoracic tract, either in the very proximal upper arm or directly in the axilla. Of course, in these situations tunneling is mandatory. When the axillary vein is punctured at the arm, tunneling is more appropriately performed so that the exit site might be located in Dawson's "green" zone (Fig. 12.4); when punctured at the axilla (typically, in children), the catheter is preferably tunneled towards the thoracic area (Figs. 12.5 and 12.6).

The advantages of PICC placement into the axillary vein are intuitive, and they have been already discussed when presenting the advantages of tunneling (reduction of infection risk and thrombotic risk; enlargement of the indication to PICCs even in patients whose basilic and brachial veins are not adequate).

12.3.2 Axillary Vein in the Infraclavicular Area

PICCs can also be inserted into the axillary vein in its thoracic tract and specifically in the infraclavicular area. This is indicated in adult patients who have specific bilateral contraindication to the cannulation of veins at the arm. The technique is

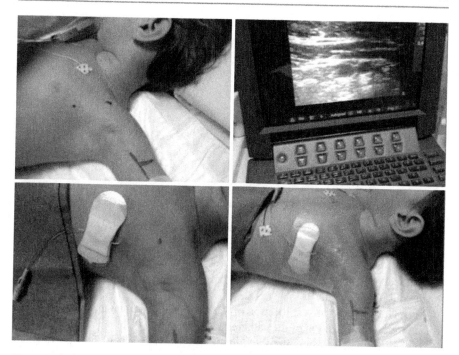

Fig. 12.5 Axillary cannulation and tunneling to the thoracic area in a child

Fig. 12.6 Axillary cannulation and tunneling to the thoracic area in a neonate

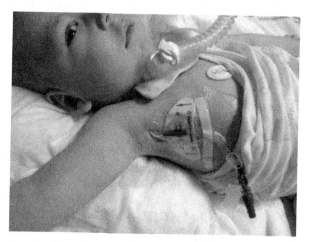

actually the same as the one described for the traditional puncture and cannulation of vein at the arm:

- Choice of a catheter of appropriate size; since the axillary vein is usually quite large in the infraclavicular area (>6 mm), this is not a critical issue: most PICC of 3-4-5 or 6Fr will fit easily.
- Ultrasound-guided venipuncture (visualization of the vein in short axis + "out-of-plane" puncture; in expert hands, visualization of the vein in long axis + "in-plane" puncture is also an option).

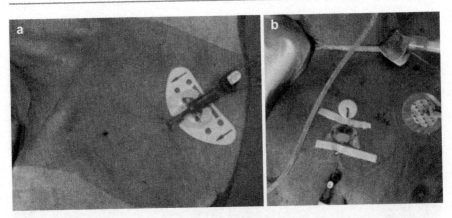

Fig. 12.7 PICCs inserted in the axillary vein, tunneled (**a**) and non-tunneled (**b**), in adults

- Modified Seldinger technique, using the micro-introducer-dilator provided in the kit.
- Ultrasound scan of the ipsilateral internal jugular vein, so as to rule out a wrong direction of the catheter.
- Verification of the correct location of the tip by the intracavitary ECG method.
- Sutureless stabilization of the catheter at the exit site.

Tunneling may be sometimes required, for instance, when the puncture site appears to be too close to the tracheostomy or to skin lesions of the infraclavicular area (Fig. 12.7).

Obvious contraindication to axillary venipuncture are morbid obesity (the vein might be far too deep), hypovolemia (the vein might be of small size or collapsed during breathing), or previous axillary/subclavian thrombosis.

The term "peripherally inserted central catheter" may not be accurate anymore in this situation, since the ultrasound-guided approach to the axillary vein is considered a direct central access. Though the "off-label" use of catheters commonly marketed as "PICCs" has many interesting clinical advantages, if compared to the use of standard CVCs:

- The micro-introducer kit provided with the PICC is particularly appropriate for axillary venipuncture, since it includes a 21G echogenic needle (less traumatic than the 18G–19G needles usually provided in the CVC kits), a floppy straight tip 0.018″ nitinol guidewire (which is the wire most likely to pass uneventfully the curve of the subclavian vein at its passage below the clavicle).
- The length of the PICC (50–60 cm) makes it ideal for any possible tunnelization, after proper trimming.
- Also, when the axillary vein is cannulated on the left side in a normal adult, the estimated length of the catheter between the exit site and the cavo-atrial junction is longer than 20–22 cm; this implies that only CVCs 25 cm long (or longer) should be used when cannulating the left axillary vein, though they might be too long when used on the right side, so that only 20 cm CVCs should be used in this case; the PICC – which can be trimmed of any desired length – has obviously a net advantage in this regard.

- Most PICCs used today are of power-injectable polyurethane, which has many advantages in terms of clinical performance [6] if compared to the standard polyurethane of most CVCs.
- PICC kits are usually equipped with many accessories (micro-introducer kit, sutureless device, needle-free connectors, etc.) which are usually absent in most CVC kits.

In our institution, the majority of central venous access for intrahospital use is achieved by PICC placement at the arm. When this is contraindicated, our second best option is the "off-label" placement of a PICC – as a direct central line – into the axillary vein in the infraclavicular area. In our clinical experience, as presented at the 2010 annual conference of AVA (Association for Vascular Access), most of these lines can be inserted by specifically trained nurses [7].

12.3.3 External Jugular Vein

The off-label insertion of PICCs in the external jugular vein in its superficial tract over the sternoclavicular muscle may be more easily accepted as an actual "peripheral insertion," since this vein is usually considered as a "peripheral" vein.

The maneuver can be performed either by ultrasound guidance or by direct puncture of the external jugular vein, which is very superficial in this tract. In children and neonates, devices based on near-infrared technology might be helpful in cannulating the vein. Considering the nonlinear trajectory of the external jugular vein, threading the catheter through this vein may be sometimes difficult. Other disadvantages are the increased risk of venous thrombosis (due to the small size of the vein) and the very uncomfortable exit site at mid-neck (unless tunneling is adopted – though tunneling may not be easy in this instance). Though, this procedure has been quite popular in recent years, since it was rapidly accepted as a "nurse-driven" procedure (i.e., insertion of a catheter in a peripheral vein) and absolutely safe, as well as requiring only limited experience in the field of vascular access [8]. A specific session of the 2008 annual conference of INS (Infusion Nursing Society) yielded an INS position paper stating that "a qualified licensed registered nurse, who is proficient in infusion therapy, may insert, care for, maintain and remove external jugular peripherally inserted central catheters (EJ-PICCs) and external jugular peripheral intravenous catheters (EJ-PIVs) [9]."

At present, the procedure is of potential interest only in the intensive care setting. In children and in adults, placement of central catheters via the axillary vein or other central veins appears to be safer and more cost-effective.

A particular approach to the external jugular vein, completely different from the one described above, is the ultrasound-guided puncture of the cannulation of the external jugular vein in its deep tract, just before its junction with the subclavian vein. This can be performed both in children and in adults, and it represents a direct central line, whose exit site (in the supraclavicular fossa) is far more convenient and comfortable than the exit site at mid-neck, though less favorable than the exit site in the infraclavicular. As such, this approach is a possible option when the axillary vein is difficult or impossible to cannulate.

12.3.4 Internal Jugular Vein

Placement of a PICC in the internal jugular vein is feasible both in children and adults, and it shares the same indications of placement in the axillary vein (i.e., local bilateral contraindications to brachial or basilic cannulation), but it is associated with an exit site in the supraclavicular fossa which is less comfortable and less desirable than an exit site in the infraclavicular area. Nonetheless, this "off-label" use of PICCs is becoming increasingly popular in the USA and the UK, since it represents the new frontier of the expansion of nurses' competence in central venous access. A 2011 Position Paper developed by AVA states that "the internal jugular veins may be considered a peripheral approach for vascular access, and are thus acceptable for cannulation by appropriately credentialed registered nurses." In the same document, PICC placement in the external jugular vein is not recommended as an option, due to the high risk of complications because of the small size of the vessel and its tortuosity [10].

The technique of PICC placement follows the same procedure as other central accesses:

- Ultrasound study of the central veins before starting the procedure (so-called RaCeVA = Rapid Central Vein Assessment)
- Ultrasound-guided puncture and cannulation, preferably with visualization of the internal jugular vein in short axis and "in-plane" venipuncture
- Modified Seldinger technique, using the micro-introducer-dilator provided in the kit
- Verification of the correct location of the tip by the intracavitary ECG method [11, 12]
- Sutureless stabilization of the catheter at the exit site

Tunnelization may be an option, especially in children, to take the catheter to an exit site below the clavicle (Fig. 12.8).

The rationale for using a PICC kit rather than a standard CVC kit is the same as described for the infraclavicular approach to the axillary vein.

12.3.5 Subclavian Vein

PICC placement in the subclavian vein is feasible, but quite uncommon. Ultrasound-guided puncture and cannulation may be performed almost exclusively by a supraclavicular approach, since the subclavian can be clearly visualized by ultrasound only by this route. The procedure might have indications in adult patients with local bilateral contraindication to PICC placement in the arm and whose internal jugular, brachiocephalic, and axillary vein may appear hard to cannulate even with ultrasound guidance.

12.3.6 Brachiocephalic Vein

Ultrasound-guided PICC placement into the brachiocephalic vein may be regarded as the first option for ultrasound-guided central venous access in neonates and small infants, as well as in children with contraindication to PICC placement in the arm [13].

Fig. 12.8 PICC inserted in the internal jugular vein (low approach) and tunneled to the infraclavicular area in an adult patient

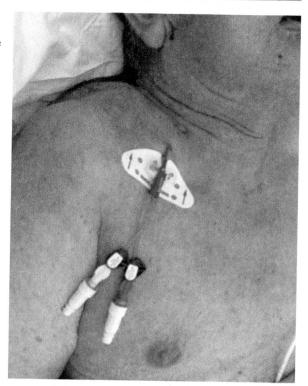

Neonates and small infants have very small peripheral veins, not suitable for ultrasound insertion of catheter 3Fr sized or larger; axillary, subclavian, and internal jugular veins have often small caliber and/or may be too risky to access. On the contrary, the brachiocephalic vein, particularly on the right side, is a very large central vein easy to puncture by ultrasound (visualization in long axis, just behind the sternoclavicular joint, and "in-plane" puncture). The risk of accidental pleural damage or arterial cannulation is minimal, and the incidence of malpositions is very low, if the proper technique is adopted [14]:

- Ultrasound bilateral scan of the central veins of the child (RaCeVA).
- Appropriate choice of a catheter size compatible with the diameter of the vein chosen for cannulation, according to the rule already discussed (3Fr catheters in 3 mm veins, 3–4Fr in 4 mm veins, 3-4-5Fr in 5 mm veins).
- Considering the small caliber of the catheters, they must preferably be made of power-injectable polyurethane, which guarantees high flow rates and optimal clinical performance; in most cases, power-injectable 3Fr single-lumen or 4Fr double-lumen PICCs are used (Fig. 12.9).
- Ultrasound-guided "in-plane" puncture of the brachiocephalic vein (puncture site close to the angle between the clavicle and the sternoclavicular muscle).
- Insertion of the catheter using the micro-introducer kit.

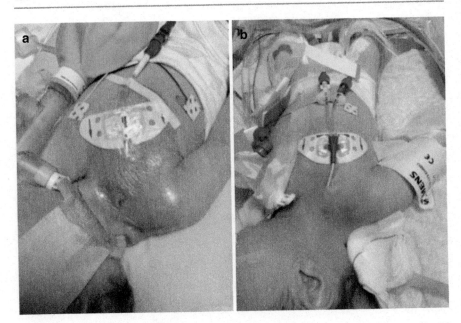

Fig. 12.9 3Fr single-lumen (**a**) and 4Fr double-lumen (**b**) power-injectable PICCs inserted in the brachiocephalic vein and tunneled to the infraclavicular area in pediatric patients

- Ultrasound control of the vein during the whole maneuver, so as to check that the guidewire and then the catheter are heading in the right direction towards the superior vena cava.
- Tunneling is always recommended; a small 3–4 cm tunnel (typically, by antero-grade tunnelization) will take the catheter to an exit site in the infraclavicular area (Fig. 12.10).
- Intra-procedural verification that the tip is at the cavo-atrial junction, using the intracavitary ECG method and/or transthoracic echocardiography.
- Securement of the catheter to the skin by suture less device; stabilization of the catheter might be improved by sealing the exit site with cyanoacrylate glue (which is also useful for closing the small incision over the puncture site, when tunneling has been performed).

The "off-label" use of PICCs for this pediatric procedure appears to be almost mandatory, considering that most pediatric CVC are characterized by an obsolete technology if compared to PICCs. Using a PICC kit allows us to choose a power-injectable catheter, to puncture the vein with a 21G echogenic needle, to cannulate the vein with a nontraumatic floppy straight tip 0.018″ nitinol guidewire, to adopt the modified Seldinger technique, and to tunnel the catheter of the desired length (since the PICC is very long and can be trimmed anywhere we want, we can make it shorter or longer depending on the estimated intravascular length and on the planned length of the tunnel). On the contrary, most pediatric CVCs are not power-injectable, their length is limited, and the kit is poor (no micro-introducer, gross needles, J-guidewire, no sutureless device, no needle-free connectors, etc.). Many

Fig. 12.10 PICC inserted in the brachiocephalic vein and tunneled to the thoracic area in a neonate; both the puncture site and the exit site are sealed with glue

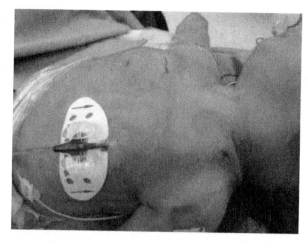

pediatric centers in Europe and the USA are currently using PICCs for this "off-label" use as CVCs. It is most likely that in the next future, the quality of the pediatric CVC will improve (adoption of more appropriate materials and accessories to achieve a safe a nontraumatic insertion).

12.3.7 Femoral Vein

PICCs are the ideal venous access device for a non-emergent access to the inferior vena cava. The contention that this is an "off-label" use may be questionable, since the femoral vein is often considered as a peripheral vein.

The main indication for this access is the presence of an obstruction of the superior vena cava or of both brachiocephalic veins (so-called superior vena cava syndrome), which implies the impossibility of using any of the abovementioned veins (brachial, basilic, axillary, internal and external jugular, subclavian, cephalic, brachiocephalic) for achieving a central access. Strictly speaking, the position of the tip inside the inferior vena cava cannot be considered as a really "central" location, the "central" location being the lower third of the superior vena cava or the upper portion of the right atrium, according to most guidelines [15]; nonetheless, there is wide consensus that a catheter whose tip is in the middle part of the inferior vena cava (above the iliac junction and below the renal veins) can be safely used for any kind of intravenous infusion, though it will be inadequate for hemodynamic monitoring.

As regards the insertion technique, tunneling is mandatory, since the exit site at the groin is associated with a very high risk of infection due to extraluminal contamination. The exit site is usually planned in the abdominal area (i.e., in the paraumbilical region or in the iliac fossa: upward tunnelization) or sometimes close to the knee (downward tunnelization).

The procedure is quite simple (Figs. 12.11, 12.12, 12.13, and 12.14) and is not associated with any relevant risk:

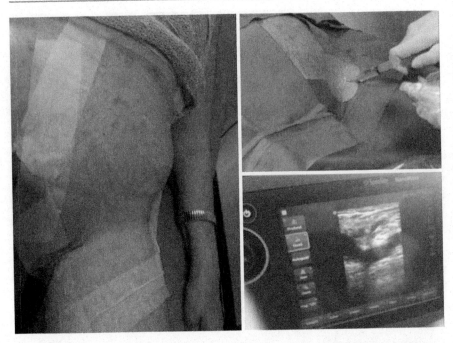

Fig. 12.11 PICC as a femoral line: ultrasound visualization of the vein before the procedure

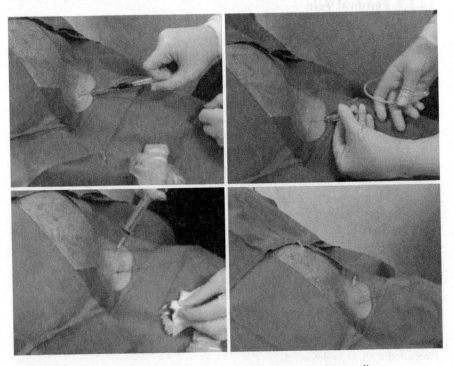

Fig. 12.12 PICC as a femoral line: venipuncture and preparation for the tunneling

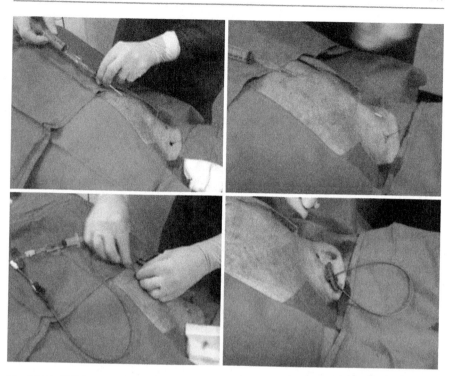

Fig. 12.13 PICC as a femoral line: anterograde tunneling using a 15 cm long 14G needle cannula

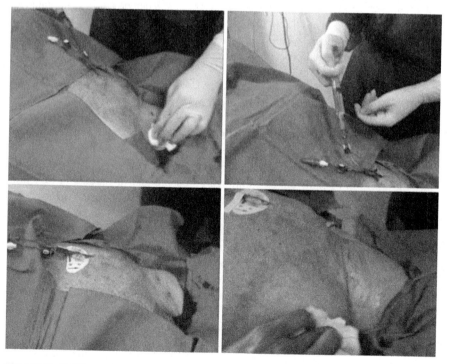

Fig. 12.14 PICC as a femoral line: final results – the incisions are all sealed with glue

- Ultrasound scan of both groins, so as to decide the best femoral vein (the catheter can be inserted either on the right or on the left side, with no differences in terms of expected complications).
- Ultrasound-guided puncture and cannulation of the femoral vein (visualization in short axis, "out-of-plane" puncture).
- Insertion of the micro-introducer-dilator.
- Trimming of the catheter to the desired length.
- Anterograde tunnelization: after proper preparation of the subcutaneous tissues with local anesthetic, the catheter is threaded through the tissues by a tunneler and then inserted into the micro-introducer.
- Securement of the catheter by sutureless device and closing all incisions with cyanoacrylate glue.

If a cuffed PICC is used (such as Pro-Line, Medcomp), the cuff should be positioned at no less than 2 cm from the exit site. The association of tunnel and cuff increases the expected duration of the device and is specifically indicated for long-term use in an extra-hospital setting.

It is noteworthy that PICCs are ideal for this type of procedure, since their considerable length (50–60 cm) is very appropriate for the catheter length required in this situation (at least 30 cm of intravascular length + at least 15–20 cm of tunnelization)

12.3.8 Saphenous Vein

PICC can also be inserted in the saphenous vein, which can be easily cannulated by ultrasound guidance in adults (in children, its caliber is too small), though the high risk of venous thrombosis which is most likely to occur when this vein is cannulated makes this a very unusual procedure.

12.4 Atypical or "Off-Label" Indication for Use

12.4.1 Apheresis, Ultrafiltration, and Dialysis

The IFU of PICCs usually consider as an appropriate clinical use of these devices only the infusion of intravenous solutions, blood product or parenteral nutrition, blood sampling, and hemodynamic monitoring. Nonetheless, in recent times PICCs have been tested also for blood-exchange procedures.

Apheresis and hemodiafiltration in critically ill pediatric patients often require a double-lumen central catheter. Considering that power-injectable double-lumen PICCs are characterized by a very high flow (1–3 ml/s), some pilot clinical studies have been performed to assess this possible "off-label" use.

In our pediatric intensive care unit, we have inserted power-injectable 5Fr double-lumen PICCs in the brachiocephalic vein (3 children: 1-, 6-, and 11-year-olds) or in the femoral vein (1 neonate, 20 days old) for the purpose of apheresis and/or

Fig. 12.15 5Fr double-lumen power-injectable PICC used for apheresis in a child with graft-vs-host disease

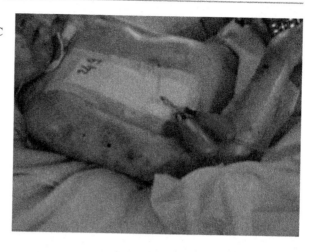

hemodiafiltration [16]. All catheters were tunneled to the infraclavicular area (if inserted in the brachiocephalic) or to the thigh. The average dwell time of the devices was 54 ± 31 days. They were used for apheresis (one patient, 6 years old, graft-vs-host disease) (Fig. 12.15) or hemofiltration (three patients, renal failure). The protocols of our institution consist in 4–6 ml/kg/min of blood flow rate and 10–20 ml/kg/h of infused fluid rate (for hemofiltration) and 1 ml/kg/min (for apheresis).

Few other reports in the literature have also investigated the possibility of using power-injectable double-lumen PICCs for apheresis, hemofiltration, and/or dialysis in pediatric patients (which usually require flow ranging from 10 to 50 ml/min) and for ultrafiltration in adults with cardiac decompensation (flow ranging from 20 to 50 ml/min).

Several factors appear to be critical and need further investigation before this use may enter the clinical practice:

- The procedure requires open-ended, non-valved power-injectable PICCs, with their unique property of allowing high flow rates.
- The tip of the catheter should be positioned in the right atrium, so as to maximize the inflow and the outflow.
- The catheter should be as short as possible (i.e., "off-label" insertion of the PICC in a central vein).
- The alarms of the apheresis/dialysis machine should be properly set.
- The procedure is more likely to be effective in neonates and children, which require limited flow rates.

References

1. Pittiruti M (2013) Central venous catheters in neonates: old territory, new frontiers. Invited commentary to Peripherally inserted central venous catheters in critically ill premature neonates, by Ozkiraz et al. J Vasc Access 14(4):318–319
2. Lamperti M, Pittiruti M (2013) Difficult peripheral veins: turn on the lights. Br J Anaesth 110(6):888–891

3. Lamperti M, Bodenham AR, Pittiruti M, Blaivas M, Augoustides JG, Elbarbary M, Pirotte T, Karakitsos D, Ledonne J, Doniger S, Scoppettuolo G, Feller-Kopman D, Schummer W, Biffi R, Desruennes E, Melniker LA, Verghese ST (2012) International evidence-based recommendations on ultrasound-guided vascular access. Intensive Care Med 38(7):1105–1117

4. Pittiruti M, Emoli A (2012) Tunnelling a PICC: when? Abstract presented at the 2012 WoCoVA – world conference on Vascular Access, Amsterdam, 26–29 June 2012

5. Dawson RB (2011) PICC Zone Insertion Method: a systematic approach to determine the ideal insertion site for PICCs in the upper arm. JAVA 16(3):156–165

6. Pittiruti M, Brutti A, Celentano D, Pomponi M, Biasucci DG, Annetta MG, Scoppettuolo G (2012) Clinical experience with power-injectable PICCs in intensive care patients. Crit Care 16(1):R21

7. Pittiruti M, Emoli A, Migliorini I, Celentano D, Scoppettuolo G (2010) Ultrasound guided infra-clavicular approach for the insertion of PICCs into the axillary vein. Abstract presented at the 2010 annual conference of AVA – Association for Vascular Access, Washington, 24–26 Sept 2010

8. Danek G, Mayer T (2001) Use of the external jugular site for PICC insertion. J Vasc Access Devices 6:14–17

9. INS – Infusion Nursing Society (2008) The role of the registered nurse in the insertion of external jugular peripherally inserted central catheters and external jugular peripheral intravenous catheters. J Infus Nurs 31(4):226–227

10. AVA – Association for Vascular Access (2011) Position statement: cannulation of the external and internal jugular veins by registered nurses and other qualified healthcare professionals. Approved by AVA Board of directors, 14 July 2011. http://www.avainfo.org/website/download.asp?id=280291

11. Pittiruti M, La Greca A, Scoppettuolo G (2011) The electrocardiographic method for positioning the tip of central venous catheters. J Vasc Access 12(4):280–291

12. Pittiruti M, Bertollo D, Briglia E, Buononato M, Capozzoli G, De Simone L, La Greca A, Pelagatti C, Sette P (2012) The intracavitary ECG method for positioning the tip of central venous catheters: results of an Italian multicenter study. J Vasc Access 13(3):357–365

13. Pittiruti M (2012) Ultrasound guided central vascular access in neonates, infants and children. Curr Drug Targets 13(7):961–969

14. Pittiruti M, Biasucci DG, Mancino A, Pulitanò S, Celentano D (2013) Ultrasound guided access to the brachio-cephalic vein in neonates, infants and small children. Abstract presented at the 2013 congress of ESPNIC – European Society of Pediatric and Neonatal Intensive Care, Rotterdam, 12–15 June 2013

15. Pittiruti M, Hamilton H, Biffi R, MacFie J, Pertkiewicz M (2009) ESPEN. ESPEN Guidelines on Parenteral Nutrition: central venous catheters (access, care, diagnosis and therapy of complications). Clin Nutr 28(4):365–377

16. Biasucci DG, Pittiruti M, Pulitanò S, Mancino A, Piastra M, Conti G (2013) Off label use of power injectable double lumen PICCs for apheresis and hemodiafiltration in neonates and children. Abstract presented at the 2013 congress of ESPNIC – European Society of Pediatric and Neonatal Intensive Care, Rotterdam, 12–15 June 2013

Venous Access Devices and Emotional Response in Oncologic Patients: Diagnostic and Management Aspects

13

Riccardo Torta and Valentina Ieraci

13.1 Introduction

The use of totally implantable venous access devices (VADs) has favorably changed the clinical management and, consequently, the quality of life (QoL) of patients requiring long-term intravenous therapy, including cancer patients. Despite their many advantages, venous access devices sometimes present functional and emotional problems. So advantages and disadvantages of the VAD from the patient's perspective should also be an important part in the selection of the type of device. The more frequent complications that arise with the use of port and tunneled catheters are physical, such as infections, thrombosis, obstructions, sleeve formation, and extravasation. But, in addition to medical issues, patients also experience psychosocial problems that can interfere with their QoL. So the patient's subjective experience of living with an implanted VAD has to be carefully considered, even if few publications discuss the psychological experience of the patient and the impact of the VADs on his or her QoL. Sometimes also excellent papers, updating the use of totally implantable venous access devices, do not discuss patient's emotional problems [30].

On the psychological point of view, we refer to the biopsychosocial model, in which to give a correct diagnosis and an effective treatment strategy for each patient, physicians face not only with the balance of physical advantages and problems of the device but also with psychological aspects, mainly represented by his or her temperament, the more or less adaptive coping style, and the emotional patient's situation. In this way, a reduction of the patient's satisfaction concerning VADs can be associated with psychosocial complaints, such as mood depression, fatigue, social impairment, and reduced QoL [16].

R. Torta (✉) • V. Ieraci
Clinical and Oncological Psychology Unit, Department of Neuroscience,
University of Turin, Via Cherasco 15, Turin 10126, Italy
email: riccardo.torta@unito.it; valentina.ieraci@unito.it

S. Sandrucci, B. Mussa (eds.), *Peripherally Inserted Central Venous Catheters,*
DOI 10.1007/978-88-470-5665-7_13, © Springer-Verlag Italia 2014

In other words, the quality of a venous access is related to the QoL through almost three dimensions: technical aspects, disease context, and patient characteristics. In this chapter, we will exclusively discuss the psychological aspects concerning the device implant in relation to the patient's emotional and cognitive characteristics.

13.2   Clinical Aspects

First of all, it is essential to define which concept of quality of life we want to refer: the health-related QoL is a meaning strictly related to a biomedical model of QoL. The physical well-being is obviously important, but QoL is a broad construct: the absence of physical symptoms does not always correspond with a complete well-being. The WHA, in 2008, coins the slogan "no health without mental health" [28]. In the same way, it is not possible to have a good QoL only considering physical aspects.

So QoL, also in patients with VADs, must be evaluated considering together the physical symptoms (related both to disease and treatments), the individual functional status (total or partial preservation of job, hobbies, daily living), the social relationships (such as interpersonal relations and social role), the well-being (e.g., compromised by anxiety, chronic stress, mood depression, and low self-esteem), and several other components (such as sexual functioning, body image, and the global patient's satisfaction). The latter is a balance between the advantages coming from the device use and the tolerability (somatic and psychological) of the same device. Such tolerability is reduced by biological complications (insertion problems, infections, thrombosis, obstructions, sleeve formation, extravasation) or by social problems (body image alterations, illness reminder linked to the device) or from psychological (discomfort, emotional symptoms, restrictions) and cognitive aspects (poor information). Anxiety and fear are common reactions in VAD patients and have been associated with realistic physical threats, such as catheter infection, thrombosis, obstruction, sleeve formation, and extravasation, but also with negative self-image and illness reminder. The most commonly reported VAD-related psychosocial problems, also in patients with home parenteral nutrition (HPN), are fatigue, depression, and social impairment, which have a major impact on patient QoL. Fatigue can be the most frequent general complaint in HPN patients and consistently interfere with daily activities such as work and leisure [15]. The National Comprehensive Cancer Network (NCCN) defines cancer-related fatigue as "a distressing persistent, subjective sense of physical, emotional and/or cognitive tiredness or exhaustion related to cancer or cancer treatment that is not proportional to recent activity and interferes with usual functioning" [22] and that is not relieved by rest [20]. This definition is according to that described by patients themselves with the addition of cognitive aspects, such as diminished concentration or attention, and emotional ones, such as distress or frustration and irritability, sleep disturbances (insomnia or hypersomnia), and decreased motivation and interest [2, 7]. Mood depression can also have a marked impact on many aspects of QoL. Huisman-de

Waal et al. [15] showed that depression was observed in 10–80 % of the HPN patients, ranging from mild to severe [16]. In our experience, about 53 consecutive patients affected by colorectal (62.5 %), lung (12.5 %), or breast (12.5 %) cancer who had their therapy performed through a port, several years ago, we found that 24.1 % of port patients showed pathological levels of mood depression (with a HADS cutoff > 8) and 20 % of subjects obtained HADS values between 6 and 7, typical of a subthreshold depression [25]. Moreover, mood depression impairs one's functional capacity to work in a social function and increases the painful physical perception [24]. Social impairment has a major impact on the daily lives, particularly in HPN patients. Huisman-de Waal et al. [15] reported that between 35 and 43 % of patients experienced social impairment due to HPN, mainly because HPN administration takes a lot of time. Moreover, VADs can interfere with social contact because of the catheter, the schedule of HPN, mobility problems, and physical complaints [15]. Both mood depression and fatigue [24] can obviously contribute to the social impairment.

13.3 Adherence Factors to Implant

The World Health Organization [28] proposed five groups of factors reducing the adherence to any kind of therapy: patient-related, condition-related, therapy-related, social-/economic-related, and healthcare team-/system-related factors. When concerning VAD implants, we will reconsider these factors under the different biopsychosocial model point of view: to evaluate the patient's adherence to a device, clinicians have to obviously consider biological aspects (such as gender, pathology, wanted side effects) but also social factors that can hardly influence patients (as the level of information and education received about the implant and the social support, from both family and medical staff, in its management). Finally, psychological factors have to be taken into account, mainly the emotional status (anxiety and particularly mood depression can increase the devices discomfort consequences and reduce the patient's motivation toward the cures), and both the temperament and the coping style can be a mainstay on the device acceptance. In this way, the temperament of an individual can strongly influence the treatment adherence: a patient that is categorized as novelty seeker at the TCI (Temperament and Character Inventory) [9] is easily inclined to accept new and also more aggressive treatments, while a harm avoider is surely more worried about possible discomforts or complications. Coping can be defined as cognitive and behavioral efforts to master, reduce, or tolerate the internal and/or external demands that are created by the stressful transaction. Coping styles are very interactive on adherence to treatments: people with a fighting spirit are more inclined to accept the negative consequences of an implant, if they can maintain an internal locus of control about the medical strategy. Patients with hopelessness are devoid of confidence in the treatment efficacy and so are more sensitive to discomfort and complications. Patients characterized by a denial coping style have great difficulty with VAD acceptance.

13.4   Evaluation Instruments

In order to evaluate the emotional status of patients that are implanted with devices, it is useful to screen the presence of anxiety, mood depression, and pathological levels of stress than can interfere with the patient's perception of the satisfaction about the devise. Other relevant aspects that have to be evaluated are the patient coping style, his or her QoL, and fatigue. It is mostly suggested to use self-evaluative instruments that allow a subjective evaluation from the patient's point of view and that are also less expensive because drawn up by patients during their permanence in the waiting rooms. If the screening cutoff is over the threshold, a standardized clinical interview takes place in order to confirm or disconfirm the screening data. An important underlying question actually was whether the occurrence of psychosocial problems associated with VAD-related complications could be somehow prevented. Fatigue severity can be measured using a subscale of the Checklist Individual Strength (CIS), composed by 8 items, with a score ranging between 8 and 56. A clinically severe fatigue can be considered present when the score is >35. This subscale demonstrated a good internal consistency and a convergent validity, with Cronbach α for fatigue severity of 0.88 [16]. Another valuation instrument for fatigue is the Edmonton Symptom Assessment System (ESAS) (Bruera et al. [5]) (0=no fatigue, 10=worse fatigue). An ESAS score ≥ 4 should be followed by an in-depth clinical evaluation, including fatigue history, physical exam, and medications, mainly in order to exclude an anemic status, vitamin deficiencies [5], and/or the usual association of CRF with a larger cluster of symptoms including sleep disturbance, emotional distress, and pain [29]. Mood depression and its severity can be evaluated with the Hospital Anxiety Depression Scale (HADS) that screens both depression and anxiety. The HADS is a 14-item (rated 0–3) self-report scale widely used in clinical practice [20]. The total HADS depression score ranges from 0 (absence of depression) to 21 (severe depression), and the proposed screening cutoff of HADS for depression is 8. Another self-evaluating instrument is the Beck Depression Inventory for Primary Care (BDI-PC) that is a 7-item self-questionnaire (each item rated 0–3) in which patients were asked to describe their past 2 weeks of symptoms. Symptoms taken into consideration are sadness, pessimism, past failure, loss of pleasure, self-dislike, self-criticalness, and suicidal thoughts and wishes. A cutoff score of >4 is given a diagnosis of major depressive disorder. The internal consistency is high ($\alpha = 0.86$), and BDI-PC was positively associated with the diagnosis of major depressive disorders ($r = 0.66$, $P < .001$) [16]. The social impairment can be carried out with the social behavior subscale of the Sickness Impact Profile 68 (SIP68) that is composed by 12 dichotomous items, with a high internal consistency (Cronbach $\alpha = 0.92$) [16]. The stress levels can be easily measured by the Distress Thermometer (DT) [12] that is a visual analog tool that asks the respondent to rate his or her level of distress in the past week on a scale from 0 (no distress) to 10 (extreme distress). The problem list (PL) consists of a list of 34 problems grouped into 5 categories (practical problems, family problems, emotional problems, spiritual/religious concerns, and physical problems) and is rated in a yes/no format. The QoL can be evaluated with EORTC or with SF 36. The EORTC QLQ-C30 [1] is composed of 30 items, concerning functional status, symptoms, and financial problems. Specific items evaluate the QoL, and the global health and single items measure specific symptoms, such as hyporexia and insomnia. Items were rated on a four-point Likert scale: "not at all, a little, quite a bit, very much." In the functional scales and in the Global Health Status, a higher score is indicative of better functioning and better QoL. To the contrary, in the symptom scales, a higher score reflects a higher level of symptoms. The Short Form (36) Health Survey [27] is a patient-reported survey of patient health that consists of eight scaled scores (vitality, physical functioning, bodily pain, general health perceptions, physical role functioning, emotional role functioning, social role functioning, and mental health). Each scale is directly transformed into a 0–100 scale on the assumption that each question carries equal weight. The lower the score, the more the disability, and the higher the score, the lesser the disability. The coping style can be evaluated with the mini-Mac that is a 29-item instrument that examines the cognitive and behavioral responses to cancer using a 4-point Likert scale. Five subscales identified fighting spirit (4 items), hopelessness (8 items), anxious preoccupation (8 items), fatalism (5 items), and cognitive avoidance (4 items) [13]. Another widespread instrument is the Brief COPE that is the abridged version of the COPE inventory and presents 14 scales all assessing different coping dimensions: active coping, planning, using instrumental support, using emotional support, venting, behavioral disengagement, self-distraction, self-blame, positive reframing, humor, denial, acceptance, religion, and substance use. Each scale contains two items (28 altogether). It can be used to assess trait coping (the usual way people cope with stress in everyday life) and state coping (the particular way people cope with a specific stressful situation) [6]. So a fast screening of emotional and distress levels can help to identify patients at risk of psychological detrimental consequences after implantation in order to support them avoiding an emotional worsening of QoL in spite of medical advantages.

13.5   Literature Data

Dearborn et al. [10] in a pivotal study compared the satisfaction with three types of permanent vascular access devices (ports, Hickman catheters, and Groshong catheters) among patients and nursing staff. Each device was associated with specific problems: patients referred fewer blood-drawing problems with port than with Groshong and Hickman but more problems with access to the device with port and more anxiety always with port. Nurses state more flow rate problems with Groshong than Hickman. However, in global satisfaction ratings, patients expressed the greatest satisfaction with port. Bow et al. [4] found no demonstrable impact of the port on the patient's QoL besides less fear of venipuncture and less pain and discomfort than experienced with a peripheral access for the administration of chemotherapy. Chernecky [8] in a reduced number of patients [21] with a VAD for chemotherapy found that patients were extremely satisfied with their VAD, particularly for decreased pain compared to venipuncture, the need for fewer needle sticks, and quicker blood draws for laboratory analysis. A third of patients referred, as negative experience, monthly heparinization, sleep disturbances, and site soreness following chemotherapy treatments. Goossens et al. [11] evaluated in a prospective study the subjective experience to have a port in daily life, and they reported that the main benefits referred by patients were no more peripheral venipuncture, greater convenience, and arms left free for activities of daily living. Nevertheless, patients disliked the visibility of ports and complained about site soreness: the negative perception of port visibility seemed to be more important to younger patients and those recently implanted. Among 106 patients with port, 69 reported that the port had no influence on their QoL, 8 patients stated a definitively positive influence of QoL, and 17 stated a definitive negative influence. The authors stressed the importance of adequate preoperative information about port: preoperative information is actually crucial for the patient and must concern a discussion of the procedure itself and what can be expected during the postoperative period. Particularly, the preoperative discussion has to deal with the advantages of no more peripheral venipuncture, no more irritating cytotoxic products through the peripheral veins, and the ability to have arms free during chemotherapy treatments. It is also very important to discuss the visibility of the port: concerning this, Lilienberg et al. [19] and Rodgers et al. [23] reported that 20 % of patients experienced problems with this factor of their treatment. We will later discuss our experience about the implication of port visibility in some kind of patients with a denial copying style. The postoperative discussion must instead be focused on the patient's education about the proper ways to recover from their surgery, how to alleviate pain when accessing the port, and to avoid lifting weights the first week after implantation. Johansson et al. [17] studied the patient's perception of having a central venous catheter or a totally implantable subcutaneous port system in 43 patients with an acute leukemia. The authors evaluated four domains (information, discomfort, anxiety, restrictions in activities). Very interesting in this study is how the patients' perception of having a central venous catheter or a totally implantable subcutaneous port system can change over time, from the day after placement to 12 weeks after placement, for example, concerning the complaint of a painful implant procedure (obviously higher near the placement) or the restrictions in daily activities that are prone to decrease over time. Globally, patients stated that the port is less restrictive in daily life than central venous catheters [17]. More recently Biffi et al. [3] evaluate 403 patients that were randomly assigned to implantation of a single type of totally implantable access port (TIAP), either through a percutaneous landmark access to the internal jugular or an ultrasound-guided access to the subclavian or a surgical cutdown access through the cephalic vein at the deltoid-pectoral groove. Patients' QoL and psychological distress were evaluated in the follow-up by EORTC QLQ-C30 and HADS questionnaires. The authors demonstrated that the different central venous insertions sites (internal jugular, subclavian, cephalic arm) were not detrimental on QoL and can contribute to lower the psychological distress [3]. Huisman-de Waal et al. [16] collected information on VAD-related physical and emotional complications from the medical charts of 110 adult HPN patients: during the observation period, there was a highly significant association (but a causal relationship) between the incidence of VAD-related complications (mainly sepsis, occlusions) and the occurrence of psychosocial complaints (depression, fatigue, social impairment, and decreased QoL). In this study, severe fatigue (CIS-fatigue score >35) was reported by 66 % of all respondents, with significant association between the degree of fatigue and the occurrence of VAD-related complications ($r=0.30$, $P=.009$); depressive disorders, evaluated with the BDI-PC, almost 57 % of the HPN patients, with a significant association between depressive disorders and both the number of experienced VAD-related problems ($r=0.30$, $P=.011$); and the number of hospital admissions due to VAD-related problems ($r=0.43$, $P=.002$). Also the social impairment evaluated with social behavior subscale of the SIP68 shows a highly significant association between social behavior, VAD-related complications ($r=0.34$, $P=.003$), and the number of hospital admissions due to VAD-related complications ($r=0.31$, $P=.026$). Low QoL was also strongly related ($P<.02$) with more intense fatigue ($r=-0.59$), more severe depression ($r=-0.68$), and greater social impairment ($r=-0.45$). There were no significant correlations between the type of venous access (AVF vs. implanted port vs. CVC) and QoL, depression, fatigue, and social impairment [16]. In our experience, port is surely an advantageous device, but in some patients, its implantation can result in emotional distress, with an increase in anxiety and depressive symptoms. This fact is linked to individual predisposition and in a more relevant sensitivity to body representation but particularly to the fact that port represents an external visible reminder of the illness. Such problem is more serious in patients that use as a coping strategy the cognitive avoidance that does not work after port implantation [25].

13.6 Therapeutic Strategies

The most important intervention on emotional problems in patients with programmed implants is prevention. Prevention can be done with a preimplant evaluation of patients' vulnerabilities concerning the background on the device and its following management. For example, psychological work could be useful on problems such as unfavorable coping style (e.g., denial or hopelessness) and a harm-avoidant temperament. Psychoeducational interventions, carried out with patients and families, can help face better cognitive and behavioral strategies about living with a VAD. Treatments of emotional problems related to the VAD implants are largely dependent on the patient's overall situation and his or her different priorities, strictly related to the stage of disease and to the symptoms induced by VADs. No studies are present concerning the specific use of these interventions on patients with VAD, and all the following statement are carried out from more general oncologic studies. Concerning fatigue, non-pharmacological interventions are mainly represented by physical therapy, such as enhanced physical activity or exercise. The goal of energy conservation is to balance rest and activities so that prioritized activities are more likely to be achieved [14]. Other interventions are represented by cognitive approaches, such cognitive behavioral therapy (CBT) or psychoeducational ones and psychosocial interventions [22]. All psychopharmacological interventions on fatigue are reported to a few different classes of drugs such as psychostimulants and antidepressants and are considered of limited effectiveness, with the exception of methylphenidate that the National Cancer Institute suggests to consider only in the treatment of severe fatigue [21]. Concerning anxiety, chronic stress, and mood depression, the class of drug of choice is antidepressants that can exert a broad activity of each of these emotional disorders. The choice of an antidepressant depends on several factors—first of all dimensional characteristics of depression, such as the particular symptomatological clusters of each patient (anhedonia, anxiety, inhibition, somatic and cognitive symptoms, etc.). But also other aspects should be taken into account: clinical and symptomatological dimensions relating to different kinds of cancer (e.g., the avoidance of antidepressants with anticholinergic activity in patients with gut motility problems in colon cancer, the avoidance of antidepressant-related prolactin increase in hormone-dependent breast cancer, the presence of uncontrolled pain that steers to the choice of antidepressants acting both on serotonin and norepinephrine); the stage of the cancer disease (an unwanted side effect, e.g., sedation, can become useful in another situation in the same patient); the risk of additional effects from antidepressant side effects and concomitant chemotherapeutic side effects (e.g., increased nausea when 5-HT antidepressants start with chemotherapy); and the pharmacodynamic and kinetic characteristics of the chosen antidepressant, particularly those concerning possible interactions with oncological drugs during polypharmacotherapeutic interventions [24].

Conclusions

A global approach to patient that has to be implanted with VADs appears a must, in order to consider also all emotional and cognitive aspects that can counteract medical advantages [26]. Only under this viewpoint is it possible to reach a full usefulness in improving the quality of life and in encouraging the autonomy of our patients.

References

1. Aronson NK, Ahmedzai S, Bergman B et al (1993) The European organization for research and treatment of cancer QLQ-C30: a quality-of-life instrument for use in international clinical trials in oncology. J Natl Cancer Inst 85:365–376
2. Barsevick A, Frost M, Zwinderman A et al (2010) On behalf of the geneqol Consortium. I'm so tired: biological and genetic mechanisms of cancer-related fatigue. Qual Life Res 19:1419–1427
3. Biffi R, Orsi F, Pozzi S et al (2011) No impact of central venous insertion site on oncology patients' quality of life and psychological distress. A randomized three-arm trial. Support Care Cancer 19:1573–1580
4. Bow EJ, Kilpatrick MG, Clinch JJ (1999) Totally implantable venous access ports systems for patients receiving chemotherapy for solid tissue malignancies: a randomized controlled clinical trial examining the safety, efficacy, costs, and impact on quality of life. J Clin Oncol 17:1267–1273
5. Bruera E, Kuehn N, Miller MJ, Selmser P, Macmillan K (1991) The Edmonton Symptom Assessment System (ESAS): a simple method for the assessment of palliative care patients. J Palliat Care 7(2):6–9
6. Carver CS (1997) You want to measure coping but your protocol's too long: consider the brief COPE. Int J Behav Med 4(1):92–100

7. Chaturvedi S, Ieraci V, Torta R (2014) Treatment of somatoform disorders and other somatic symptom condition (pain, fatigue, hot flashes, pruritus). In: Grassi L, Riba M (eds) Psychopharmacology in oncology and palliative care – a practical manual. Springer, Germany
8. Chernecky C (2002) Satisfaction versus dissatisfaction with venous access devices in outpatient oncology: a pilot study. Oncol Nurs Forum 29(7):1029–1030
9. Cloninger CR, Przybeck TR, Svrakic DM (1991) The Tridimensional Personality Questionnaire: U.S. normative data. Psychol Rep 69:1047–1057
10. Dearborn P, De Muth JS, Requarth AB et al (1997) Nurse and patient satisfaction with three types of venous access devices. Oncol Nurs Forum 24(1 Suppl):34–40
11. Goossens GA, Vrebos M, Stas M et al (2005) Central vascular access devices in oncology and hematology considered from a different point of view. J Infus Nurs 28:61–67
12. Grassi L, Johansen C, Torta R et al, on behalf of the Italian Society of Psycho-Oncology Distress Thermometer Study Group (2013) Screening for distress in cancer patients. A multicenter, nationwide study in Italy. Cancer 119 (9):1714–1721
13. Grassi L, Torta R, Varetto A et al (2005) Styles of coping with cancer: the Italian version of the Mini-Mental Adjustment to Cancer (Mini-MAC) scale. Psychooncology 14(2):115–124
14. Howell D, Keller-Olaman S, Oliver TK et al (2013) A pan-Canadian practice guideline and algorithm: screening, assessment, and supportive care of adults with cancer-related fatigue. Curr Oncol 20(3):e233–e246
15. Huisman-de Waal G, Schoonhoven L, Jansen J et al (2007) The impact of home parenteral nutrition on daily life-a review. Clin Nutr 26:275–288
16. Huisman-de Waal G, Versleijen M, van Achterberg T et al (2011) Psychosocial complaints are associated with venous access-device related complications in patients on home parenteral nutrition. JPEN J Parenter Enteral Nutr 35(5):588–595
17. Johansson E, Engervall P, Björvell H et al (2009) Patients' perceptions of having a central venous catheter or a totally implantable subcutaneous port system – results from a randomised study in acute leukaemia. Support Care Cancer 17:137–143
18. Kearns NP, Cruickshank CA, McGuigan KJ et al (1982) A comparison of depression rating scales. Br J Psychiatry 141:45–49
19. Lilienberg A, Bengtsson M, Starkhammar H (1994) Implantable devices for venous access: nurses' and patients' evaluation of three different port systems. J Adv Nurs 19(1):21–28
20. Mitchell SA, Beck SL, Hood LE et al (2007) Putting evidence into practice: evidence-based interventions for fatigue during and following cancer and its treatment. Clin J Oncol Nurs 11:99–113
21. National Cancer Institute (NCI) (2013) United States, National Institutes of Health, Fatigue (PDQ). Health Professional Information [Web page]. NCI, Bethesda
22. National Comprehensive Cancer Network (2009) NCCN clinical practice guidelines in oncology: cancer-related fatigue. Ver. 2.2009. NCCN, Fort Washington
23. Rodgers HC, Liddle K, Nixon SJ et al (1998) Totally implantable venous access devices in cystic fibrosis: complications and patients' opinions. Eur Respir J 12(1):217–220
24. Torta RG, Ieraci V (2013) Depressive disorders and pain: a joint model of diagnosis and treatment. J Pain Relief S2. http://dx.doi.org/10.4172/2167-0846.S2-003
25. Torta R, Varetto A, Binaschi L (2006) Emotional problems in patients with totally implantable venous access system (PORT). Psychooncology 15(S2):445
26. Torta R, Varetto A, Sandrucci S et al (2000) Totally implantable venous systems (port) and quality of life. Ann Oncol 11(2):29
27. Ware JE, Sherbourne CD (1992) The MOS 36-item short-form health survey (SF-36). I. Conceptual framework and item selection. Med Care 30(6):473–483
28. World Health Organization (2008) Millennium Development Goal 5 – improving maternal health. WHO
29. Xiao C (2010) The state of science in the study of cancer symptom clusters. Eur J Oncol Nurs 14:417–434
30. Zaghal A, Khalife M, Mukherji D et al (2012) Update on totally implantable venous access devices. Surg Oncol 21:207–215

Peripheral Inserted Central Catheters: Medicolegal Aspects

14

Rita Celli

Let us get started with a dichotomy that needs to be clear: the *fil rouge* that joins law and medicine together.

Medical jurisprudence: deals with legal aspects of medical practice of doctors.

Forensic medicine: deals with medical aspects of law and medicolegal case management.

This work will take into account the first issue.

The threat of clinical negligence litigation for responsibility[1] remains a great apprehension for all practicing doctors since there has been a steady rise in the number of claims for negligence in the last years.

Doctors have the statutory duty to maintain and continuously improve clinical standards through clinical governance. Despite this, standards sometimes fall, and patients more often turn to the courts for remuneration.

The legal standard of care is currently a professionally based standard determined by the evidence provided by expert witnesses. The adoption of *guidelines* in clinical practice has been increasing with the aim to help standardize care all over the world. There may be a role for the use of guidelines in determining the legal standard of care, which could improve healthcare quality and reduce harm to patients.

---

[1] *Responsibility*

Accountability, the condition of being required to account for one's actions

Corporate social responsibility, a set of generally accepted relationships, obligations, and duties that relate to an institution's impact on the welfare of society

Miller-Keane Encyclopedia and Dictionary of Medicine, Nursing, and Allied Health, Seventh Edition. © 2003 by Saunders, an imprint of Elsevier, Inc.

All rights reserved.

R. Celli
Studio Medico-legale Viglino, Corso G. Ferraris 147, Turin, Italy
e-mail: ritacelli.sml@gmail.com

S. Sandrucci, B. Mussa (eds.), *Peripherally Inserted Central Venous Catheters*,
DOI 10.1007/978-88-470-5665-7_14, © Springer-Verlag Italia 2014

We can easily point out five events that might alert the physician to impending litigation:

1. A clear error is made.
2. A serious and unexpected accident occurs in the course of treatment.
3. The patient is clearly dissatisfied. Many legal actions are commenced by discontent patients who feel their physician did not give them enough attention; these patients may then attribute a result that is less than perfect to the carelessness of the physician rather than being an acceptable complication.
4. A complaint is made to the law authority.
5. A self-rule decision is made by the law authority to hold an inquest or investigation into the death of a patient.

The most common notice of an impending legal action is the receipt of a letter from a lawyer on behalf of the patient or from the law enforcing agencies. Some of these letters (those from the lawyer) simply request copies of the medical records and may include general questions for the physician about the treatment rendered, the complication that occurred, and the current prognosis for the patient.

A good working knowledge of the law in this regard, coupled with a thorough understanding of the correct method of dealing with such cases, helps one to build confidence over riding the fear of responsibility.

14.1 The Violation of Contract

Almost all over the world these claims are made when it is alleged that the physician has breached an expressed or implied term of the agreement that arises out of the physician-patient relationship, usually an allegation that the physician failed to achieve the guaranteed result. A claim for violation of contract is also advanced when it is alleged that the physician has disclosed confidential information about the patient without proper authorization and in the absence of being required to disclose the information by law. In Italy, the concept of the medical contract has a general application where a direct physician-patient relationship has been established. The existence of a medical contract does not necessarily impose an obligation of result to the physician, although the physician may have an obligation of means.

14.2 Informed Consent

It is now widely accepted that clinicians should negotiate rather than dictate what is in the best interests of patients.

Several decades ago, it was common for clinicians to minimize the importance of respecting the autonomy of patients in clinical practice, their ability, and need to make plans about the personal consequences of treatment for them and others.

It is not unusual today for a claim to be asserted on behalf of the plaintiff alleging that, in obtaining consent, the physician failed to provide all the information about the nature and anticipated effect of the proposed procedure, including the significant risks and possible alternatives that a reasonable person would wish to know in determining whether to proceed. The notion of informed consent is entrenched in many codes of ethics and in legislation, in Italy particular in the Civil Code, and gives the tools in current professional and legal guidance about obtaining informed consent from competent patients.

> Successful relationships between doctors and patients depend on trust. To establish that trust, patients' autonomy must be respected. They must be given sufficient information, in a way that they can understand, in order to enable them to make informed decisions about their care.

For example, in England a wide range of professional organizations—including the British Medical Association, the Royal Colleges, and the various defense associations—all endorse the same moral principles.

The same can be said of professional and regulatory bodies in other countries.

The law also endorses the moral importance of respect for autonomy within medicine. To avoid a claim of battery, the consent of patients to treatment must be based on information "in broad terms" about the nature of, and reason for, proposed treatment choices. Separate consent must be provided for distinct procedures. Patients should be informed about which procedures within a treatment plan are independent and consent obtained for each component therapy, rather than for the plan as if it were as an indistinguishable whole. This will be so, even if refusal of one component may seriously compromise the patient's prospects for recovery.

The new standards were worrisome for physicians, creating great uncertainty about what was expected of them. It would appear, however, that physicians have come to appreciate the need for more detailed explanations to be given to their patients and are finding the requirements of informed consent are not imposing as stringent a hardship as once feared. The successful defense of such actions is assisted by the overriding requirement, that to succeed the plaintiff must demonstrate that in the face of full disclosure, a reasonable person in the patient's place would have refused the procedure.

There is a very basic proposition recognized by the courts all over the world that every human being of adult years and of sound mind has the right to determine what shall be done with his or her own body. This general principle is that of the inviolability of the person mostly in all countries. Therefore, subject to certain exceptions, such as an emergency or a court order, a physician must obtain a valid and informed consent before any treatment is administered to a patient.

An emergency nullifying the requirement to obtain consent only exists where there is imminent and serious danger to the life or health of the patient and it is necessary to proceed immediately to treat the patient. The concept of emergency treatment also extends to instances where the patient requires treatment to alleviate severe suffering. The convenience of the physicians, the healthcare team, and the hospital, however, must not be included as determining factors in declaring proposed treatment to be emergent.

The following suggestions may help physicians meet the legal standards applicable to the law of consent:

- Discuss with the patient the nature and anticipated effect of the proposed treatment, including the significant risks and available alternatives.
- Give the patient the opportunity to ask questions.
- Tell the patient about the consequences of leaving the ailment untreated. Although there should be no appearance of coercion by unduly frightening patients who refuse treatment, the courts now recognize there is a positive obligation to inform patients about the potential consequences of their refusal.
- Be alert to and deal with each patient's concerns about the proposed treatment. It must be remembered that any patient's special circumstances might require disclosure of potential although uncommon hazards of the treatment when ordinarily these might not seem relevant.
- Exercise cautious discretion in accepting waivers, even if the patient waives all explanations, has no questions, and may be prepared to submit to the treatment whatever the risks.

In order to avoid a claim of negligence, the information disclosed to patients, when obtaining consent about risks, must be "reasonable" in the eyes of the court, leaving aside breaches of professional duty so obvious that they "speak for themselves." The care is regarded as appropriate if the experts convince the court that a relevant reasonable body of professional opinion would endorse the course of action that was actually taken. In the case of consent, the issue would be the amount and accuracy of information disclosed by a doctor and contested by a patient.

Being short of suitable action of this will be irrespective of:

1. The degree that claimants believe that they were morally entitled to specific information they were not given
2. The degree of harm they suffered as a result

Consent assessed as appropriate is judged by a "professional standard" which may be inappropriate outside the profession if it disregards the patient and is based solely on the views of clinicians.

In the past, some patients were not given the information about therapeutic risks when they clearly should have been. Such moral breaches of the duty to respect the patient's autonomy have recently led the judiciary to question the relevance of the appropriate standard for determining what patients should be told about risks.

When faced with a decision about how much information to reveal, the most morally appropriate behavior is not to speculate about what expert colleagues might do but rather to ask what a "reasonable person" would wish to know in the circumstances of the patient. In practice, this should be interpreted, as meaning what clinicians themselves would wish to know in similar circumstances.

Furthermore, the moral and legal acceptability of consent depends upon more than the transmission of appropriate information to patients. Their choices must not be coerced by members of their healthcare team or by others (e.g., relatives). Equally, patients must be competent to consent: to be able to understand, remember, deliberate about, and believe clinical information given to them about their specific treatment options. Competence is task oriented: patients should not be thought of as either totally competent or incompetent. Judgments about competence to consent should depend on the particular circumstances involved.

Both professional guidance and legal precedent reinforce these provisions for valid consent. In general the clinical duty to obtain proper informed consent is now widely believed to be an essential component of good clinical practice.

Some clinicians have found it difficult to embrace this professional and legal consensus. They argue that in some clinical circumstances, competent patients may feel unable to understand the information they require to give proper consent. Of course, if patients are incompetent, then the issue of consent does not arise.

Empirical research suggests that the understanding of patients improves with the provision of information structured according their needs and with the use of a variety of strategies for good communication. Not surprisingly, poor communication may lead to poor understanding.

In the context of informed consent, this fact in itself does not constitute evidence that reduces the moral importance of relevant information disclosure. Again, the communication skills of clinical researchers doing this kind of work will be important when conclusions are drawn about good practice.

The fact that patients may say that they want their clinicians to make final decisions about their care does not mean that they do not want to be involved in it. In fact, such patients may be simply be stating the obvious—that clinicians must still make the final decision to proceed with treatment after informed consent has been given. Obviously care should be taken from drawing the wrong conclusions from interviews with distressed patients who may feel intimidated and less than honest about their real feelings.

14.3   Negligence, Malpractice, and Civil Liability

The majority of legal actions brought against physicians are based on a claim for negligence or malpractice. These actions involve an allegation that the defendant physician did not exercise a reasonable and acceptable standard of care, competence, and skill in attending upon the patient and, as a result, the patient suffered harm or injury.

Courts have long recognized that the physician-patient relationship is built on trust; this relationship of trust is recognized in the concept of fiduciary duty. Physicians' fiduciary duty means they must act with good faith and loyalty toward the patient and never place their own personal interests ahead of the patient's. Fiduciary duty may be asserted regarding any duty imposed by law arising from the physician-patient relationship. The hallmarks of a fiduciary duty are:
- An imbalance of power between the parties (often found by courts to exist between doctors and patients)
- An ability in the stronger party to affect the weaker party's interests
- A particular vulnerability on the part of the weaker party

14.4   Professional Distortion, Liability

The elements of negligent misrepresentation include a special or professional relationship between the parties; the representation or opinion must be untrue, inaccurate, or misleading due to the negligence of the professional; the receiver must have relied on the misrepresentation or erroneous opinion; and as a result of such reliance, the patient must have suffered damages. When providing a medicolegal report or expert opinion, physicians must take care to remain within their area of practice or specialty and avoid vague statements or speculation as to prognosis.

According to the Italian penal code, individuals are personally liable for negligent acts or malpractice they commit (direct liability). Individuals may not be held liable for the negligence or malpractice of their agents. So, in Italy, the so-called vicarious liability does not exist.

It follows that physicians may not be held liable for the work of any health professional in their employment. A physician who practices in a partnership is not jointly liable for negligent acts or malpractice committed by any partner in the course of the partnership business.

In the hospital setting, the hospital is vicariously liable for the negligent acts or malpractice of nurses, physiotherapists, and other healthcare providers it engages as employees or agents of the hospital. Physicians on the medical staff of a hospital are engaged as dependent contractors and employees. There is therefore vicarious liability on the hospital for the negligence or malpractice of physicians on the medical staff.

14.5   Heads of Departments and Chiefs of Staff

Physicians are potentially liable when accepting positions as head of a department or chief of staff. There have been some legal actions where the role of a physician as head of a department or chief of staff has been a focal point in the litigation. This is not to say there is more risk of liability, rather it is to put the magnitude of the risk in perspective.

As head of a department or chief of staff, physicians function as officers of the hospital. The duties extend to the selection, organization, and monitoring of both professional and nonprofessional staff, as well as the acquisition and maintenance of appropriate facilities and equipment to reasonably ensure that patients receive adequate and proper care.

The specific duties and responsibilities of heads of departments and chiefs of staff are often set out in the hospital's bylaws. Generally, physicians in these positions are expected to:

(a) Exercise responsibility for the general clinical organization of the hospital.
(b) Supervise all professional care given to all patients within the hospital.
(c) Report to the medical committee respecting medical diagnosis, care, and treatment provided to the patients of the hospital.
(d) Exercise responsibility for the organization and implementation of clinical review programs and encourage continuing medical education.

(e) Get involved in the management of the patient when becoming aware that a serious problem in diagnosis, care, or treatment exists and appropriate steps have not being taken by the attending physician.

Sometimes there is fear that the head of a department or the chief of staff might be held responsible for any mishaps caused by any other member of the medical staff or any other healthcare provider over whom it may be said they have administrative or supervisory responsibilities. It is always difficult to speculate about the extent to which legal liability might devolve in any hypothetical situation. Much depends on the circumstances of each case. Nevertheless, the head of a department or the chief of staff is not expected to be a guarantor of the work of other members of the medical staff or other healthcare providers.

More specifically, the liability of heads of departments or chiefs of staff does not extend to their being held liable simply for the negligence or malpractice of some other member of the medical staff or other healthcare providers. Liability is only engaged if they fail to act reasonably in carrying out the duties assigned to them by legislation and the bylaws of the hospital or if they fail to intervene when they know, or ought to know, that a patient may come to harm without intervention.

14.6 Incidence of Legal Actions

There has been a steady increase in the number of legal actions brought against physicians. This is thought to be due in part to worst medical care resulting in adverse events, even if it is clear that physicians increased awareness and understanding of patient safety measures and enhanced risk management procedures.

Let us summarize the factors again which contribute to the commencement of a legal action against a physician:

- There has been a change in public attitude toward the fallibility of the physician. Patients are more often likely to consider that any complication or unsatisfactory result was avoidable in spite of the best efforts of the physician.
- Public awareness of recent advances in medicine often leads to unrealistic expectations such that people connect complications and poor results with negligent treatment.
- Counsel for the patient may be encouraged to initiate or continue with some legal actions due to an unrealistic standard of care advocated by expert consultants retained on behalf of the patient.
- The most frequent factor is a lack of adequate communication between the physician and the patient.

14.7 The Expert Consultant

The expert consultant assists and advises the court through the expression of expert opinion as to what constitutes a reasonable standard of conduct, skill, and knowledge in the circumstances of a particular case. Above all else, the expert is expected to be impartial. It is not the role of the expert to act as an advocate for any party.

Physicians asked to act, as an expert consultant must honestly self-evaluate whether they are appropriately qualified to provide the necessary opinion in the circumstances of that case. The potential expert may feel that another physician of greater or different experience, or another specialty, is more suitable to assess the work. Physicians should not fall into the trap of believing that only leading specialists are qualified to act as expert consultants. In fact, an experienced general practitioner is best qualified to speak of the work of another general practitioner.

The expert must be guided by personal experience and what is perceived to be the usual or acceptable practice of colleagues in similar circumstances. Careful consideration must also be given to the education, experience, and other qualifications of the defendant physician, as well as to the equipment, facilities, and other resources that were available. It has been suggested that, as a final check, the expert consultant should ask whether the complication or result may have happened to any other physician even when being reasonably careful. If so, the defendant physician should not be considered to have been in breach of the appropriate duty of care toward the patient.

The expert consultant should remember that, in formulating an opinion about the quality of past medical care, it is a luxury to be able to review all the facts in retrospect. Allowances must be made to adjust for this advantage. It is equally important for the expert consultant to ensure the work of the physician is assessed according to the standards of practice applicable at the time of the event. The standards of practice change quickly, and it would be unfair to review the work of the physician in the light of later practice.

14.8   Negligence, Malpractice, and the Standard of Care

It has often been said that medicine is not an exact science and that a physician does not guarantee satisfactory results or the patient's renewed good health. Problematic results may occur in medical procedures even when the highest degrees of skill and care have been applied. Taking for granted that the law does not demand perfection, there is a standard of care that a physician must exercise in order not to be considered negligent.

Consistently over the years, the majority of medicolegal actions brought against physicians have been based on a claim for negligence or malpractice. Allegations of negligence or malpractice extend not only to acts the physician is said to have committed in error but also to steps suggested the physician should have taken but failed to take. Indeed, this latter category, the alleged omission on the part of the physician, constitutes the bulk of claims for negligence or malpractice.

Four elements must be established or proven for any legal action based upon a claim for negligence to be successful:

1. There must be a duty of care owed toward the patient.
2. There must be a violation of that duty of care.
3. The patient must have suffered harm or injury.
4. The harm or injury must be *directly related* (casual connection) to the breach of the duty of care.

In Italian law, it is established that the *duty of care* imposed on a physician arises naturally out of the physician-patient relationship. This duty arises out of the principles of general civil liability (civil code), substantially altogether with the penal code. Accepting a patient creates a duty, an obligation, to attend to the patient as the situation requires and as circumstances reasonably permit. The physician also has an obligation to make a diagnosis and to advise the patient of it. The physician is not expected to be correct every time, rather they are merely expected to exercise reasonable care, skill, and judgment in arriving at a diagnosis.

Another duty imposed by the physician-patient relationship requires the physician to properly treat the patient in accordance with the current and accepted standards of practice (guidelines). Further, the physician has an obligation to refer the patient or to obtain consultation when unable to diagnose the patient's condition, when the patient is not responding to treatment, or when the required treatment is beyond the competence or experience of the physician. In the same vein, referral or coverage arrangements must be made when the physician is not available to continue treatment the patient. There is also a duty upon physicians to adequately instruct patients about both active treatment and follow-up care. This applies not only to return appointments and referrals for lab tests or consultations but also to clinical signs and symptoms that might signal a complication requiring the patient to seek immediate medical care.

In determining whether a physician has breached a duty of care toward a patient, the courts consider the standard of care and skill that might reasonably have been applied by a colleague in similar circumstances. In particular every medical practitioner must bring to his task a reasonable degree of skill and knowledge and must exercise a reasonable degree of care. He is bound to exercise that degree of care and skill which could reasonably be expected of a normal, prudent practitioner of the same experience, and standing and, if he regards himself as a specialist, a higher degree of skill is required of him.

The appropriate measure is therefore the level of reasonableness and not a standard of perfection. The courts have also recognized that it is easy to be wise in hindsight; therefore, they must guard against judging a physician in retrospect. In addition, legal actions often take years to arrive to trial, and medical standards may have changed in the interim. It is important that the appropriate standard be determined with reference to the circumstances and the reasonable standard of care as it applied at the time of the alleged negligence. The court ascertains this reasonable standard by means of expert evidence at trial.

It has long been held that physicians are not in breach of their duty toward a patient simply because they have committed an honest error of judgment after a careful examination and thoughtful analysis of a patient's condition. The courts have attempted to distinguish an error of judgment from an act of carelessness due to a lack of knowledge.

It must be established that there is a relationship, or causal connection, between the alleged breach of duty and the stated harm or injury. This issue often becomes the core of a legal action. Until recently, in Italy, when the cause of the complication was not readily evident, counsel for the plaintiff would attempt to bridge the gap by resorting to the maxim res ipsa loquitur or "the thing speaks for itself." The Supreme Court has recently stated that using this maxim to establish causation is inappropriate. Medical science has not yet reached the stage where the law ought to presume that all treatment afforded to a patient must have a successful outcome and that anything less suggests negligence or malpractice. The scientific criteria must be applied with a serious probability (very close to 100 %) that a different kind of standard of care would have made the very difference in the outcome.

Suggested Reading

Doyal L (2009) Good clinical practice and informed consent are inseparable. Heart 87(2):103–6
Faden RR, Beauchamp TL (1986) A history and theory of informed consent. Oxford University Press, New York
Shanmugam K (2002) SMA lecturer 2001: testing the Bolam test: consequences of recent developments. Singapore Medical J 43(1):7–11

Judgements According to Italian Law

Corte di Cassazione, Sect. 5, Sentence n. 45801 17/09/2008 Ud. (dep. 11/12/2008) Rv. 242207 President Ambrosini G, Compiler Federico R, Reporting Judge Federico R, Public Proceeder Monetti V
Corte di Cassazione, Sect. 4. Sentence n. 11335 16/01/2008 Cc (dep. 14/03/2008) Rv. 238967. President Marini L, Compiler Piccialli P, Reporting Judge Piccialli P, Public Proceeder Iannelli M
Corte di Cassazione, Sect. 4. Sentence n. 37077 24/06/2008 (dep. 30/09/2008) Rv. 240963. President Licari C, Compiler Piccialli P, Reporting Judge Piccialli P, Public Proceeder Bua FM
Corte di Cassazione, Unified Sect. U, Sentence n. 2437 18/12/2008 Ud. (dep. 21/01/2009) Rv. 241752. President Gemelli T, Compiler Macchia A, Reporting Judge Macchia A, Public Proceeder Ciani G
Corte di Cassazione, Sect. 4. Sentence n. 21799 20/04/2010 Ud. (dep. 08/06/2010) Rv. 247341. President Mocali P, Compiler Massafra U. Reporting Judge Massafra U, Public Proceeder Stabile C
Corte di Cassazione, Sect. 4. Sentence n. 37077 24/06/2008 Ud. (dep. 30/09/2008) Rv. 240963. President Licari C. Compiler Piccialli P. Reporting Judge Piccialli P. Public Proceeder Bua FM

Judgements According to British Law

Bolam v Friern Hospital Management Committee (1957) I WRL 582
Barnett v Chelsea & Kensington Hospital (1968) I All ER 1068; Whitehouse v Jordan (1981) I All ER 267; Sidaway v Bethlem Royal Hospital Governors (1985) AC 871; Maynard v West Midlands Health Authority (1985) I All ER 635; Bolitho v City and Hackney Health Authority (1997) 4 All ER 771; Palmer v Tees Health Authority (1998) All ER 180 and (1999) Lloyd's Medical Reports 151 (CA)

The PICC Team

15

Kathryn Ann Kokotis

15.1 History

The procedure of peripheral IV cannulation shifted from being a doctor-dominated procedure to being a nurse-dominated procedure in the 1970s. Massachusetts General Hospital in Boston was the first to allow a nurse, ADA Plummer RN, to administer IV therapy and she became the first IV nurse who also formed the first IV team [33]. On another front, the world was changing in terms of vascular access and long line or PICC line insertion. The origination of the PICC team (Peripherally Inserted Central Catheter team) is historically unclear. Anecdotal commentary follows that the very first nursing-based long line, a precursor to the PICC (Peripherally Inserted Central Catheter) line was placed in the 1970s. The first anecdotal nursing team to place a PICC line (long line) was at MD Anderson Cancer Center, at the University of Texas (Houston), in the United States. The time period was the 1970s and the nurses involved were Millie Lawson RN, the IV Team Manager and Suzanne Herbst RN, a medical consultant. The application for PICC lines or long lines was for the oncology patient receiving chemotherapeutic drugs in the hospital and outpatient center. At what point did the concept of a PICC team evolve is still somewhat of a mystery. Nursing intravenous therapy teams (IV teams) were established throughout the early 1970s and 1980s; however, their primary function was to place peripheral intravenous catheters (PIVs), administer infusion medications, perform tubing changes and dressing changes, as well as act as a resource for the clinical staff. Scattered throughout the world from the 1970s to present are clinicians,

Financial disclosure: Kathy Kokotis is an employee of Bard Access Systems. Stock holdings include CR Bard and Johnson and Johnson.
Background: Kathy Kokotis has been in vascular access for over 25 years. Past history includes serving as Director of Infection Control.

K.A. Kokotis, RN, BS, MBA
Director, Global Clinical Education for Bard Access Systems,
936 Cornwallis Lane, Munster, IN 46321, USA
e-mail: Kathy.kokotis@crbard.com

S. Sandrucci, B. Mussa (eds.), *Peripherally Inserted Central Venous Catheters*,
DOI 10.1007/978-88-470-5665-7_15, © Springer-Verlag Italia 2014

especially nurses, who place what were termed long lines or now PICC lines composed of silicone or polyurethane. These clinicians are sometimes part of an IV team, PICC team, or are independent practitioners in various units of the hospital setting that do not necessarily belong to a dedicated team or process. This leads to the question of what is an actual PICC team and how do they function?

15.2 Definition of the PICC Team

The evolution of the PICC line placer in essence is multifaceted. PICC line placers come in various structures and form. They may be part of a full service team such as an IV team or they may be part of a team that concentrates on PICC line placement and care alone, or they may be individuals that are scattered throughout the facility that perform services on an as-needed basis. Lastly, a PICC placer may be an outside agent that is contracted to place PICC lines in a facility. Not all of these constitute a PICC line team. A team is defined as a group of individuals with a set of complementary skills required to complete a task, job, or project. Team members are accountable for collective performance and work towards common goals with shared rewards. A team is more than a collection of individuals when a strong sense of mutual commitment creates synergy, thus generating performance greater than the sum of the performance of an individual member [13]. This leads to the question: is a lone PICC placer a proceduralist or a team? By the definition of a team, who places PICC lines alone is likely a proceduralist.

The outside contractual agent or service that is hired to place PICC lines in various types of facilities is composed of independent contracted clinicians. Each clinician acts as a sole agent and is accountable for their own individual performance. In this type of setting, it is difficult to work towards a common goal or outcomes, as one is hired to perform the function on an as-needed basis. In this scenario, the clinician acts as a hired gun to perform procedural tasks. These tasks include line placement, line removal, dressing change, declotting, and potentially line troubleshooting, for a contractual fee. The disadvantage of this type of system lies in the fact that the line is not necessarily placed within hours of a physician order or even the same day, thus potentially delaying medication delivery. The days of a PICC line not being an urgent procedure in today's healthcare may be a misnomer. As we match the vascular access device to the patient for safety and efficacy, the PICC line becomes an important part of the vascular access arsenal. Delayed placement contributes to delayed therapy and potentially alters patient outcomes. In the case of a contractual agency, the facility is relying on the contractual service to monitor the competency of its outside clinical agents and their adherence to guidelines on infection prevention. In today's climate, ownership of outcomes and data is becoming paramount to prevention strategies. On the other hand, if a facility cannot maintain the competency of clinicians to place PICC lines or afford the financial labor for a full-time employee, a contractual agency may provide a valuable service. Davis and Kokotis [16] indicate that an outside contractor may guarantee insertion success of 90–100 % but does not guarantee outcomes related to complications. Some agencies may monitor complication rates and provide reporting to the payer. Lastly, with a contractual agency, it is difficult to implement early patient assessment for the best vascular access device to complete therapy. As contractual agencies are called on an as-needed basis, they are often called when the vascular access is completely exhausted.

The same is true of training nurses throughout the facility to place PICC lines on an as-needed basis. This process is defined by Hornsby et al. [23] as the "PICC, Stick, and Run Team" concept. Covenant Healthcare System in Saginaw, Michigan, implemented this type of system in the early 1990s without success. The facility trained 30 nurses, in various units over an eight year period to place PICC lines as needed. Training consisted of a didactic with a practicum. The next step in training post didactic and practicum was the observation of successful insertions with a proctor. Between the time period of 1990 and 1998, 30 nurses were trained at a cited training cost of $33,000. Of the 30 nurses trained from various units to place PICC lines, on an as-needed basis, only 4 nurses achieved a minimum competency level with proctoring. This training cost resulted in an additional $340 to the placement of each of the 97 PICC lines placed in 1997 alone. As a result, the majority of PICC line placements continued to be sent to the Interventional Radiology Department, which, though costly, maintained a higher success rate for placement. The hospital found themselves in a continuous loop of training and retraining clinical staff, and only 10 % of their clinicians achieved minimum competency post proctoring. The additional problem with a "PICC, Stick, and Run Team" is being able to supply the labor time to place a PICC line on demand. It becomes impossible to ask clinical staff or supervisory staff to allocate 1–2 h of the day for the placement of a PICC line. In addition, asking a clinician who only performs PICC line placements once a week, once a month, or once a year to be able to maintain the competency level needed for successful outcomes is a difficult proposition. At Covenant Healthcare System, the "PICC, Stick, and Run Team" concept was replaced with a dedicated full-time PICC team in 2001, comprised of three nurses placing over 2,000 PICC lines a year, in an approximately 500-bed facility.

The traditional IV teams have dedicated staffing and have the goal of working in conjunction with other members of the team to facilitate patient outcomes related to vascular access. These teams are traditionally involved in the placement of PIVs, PICC lines, and midlines as well as the care and maintenance of devices. They also provide education to clinical staff members, on infection prevention and troubleshooting. As many of these traditional teams started with the placement of PIVs, it becomes difficult for these teams to become focused on the vascular access assessment decision of the proper vascular access device to meet the patient's therapy. Time constraints in daily duties of PIV placement can become overwhelming. These teams can find themselves becoming procedural teams rather than vascular access planning teams. On the other hand, the dedicated PICC teams which focus solely on PICC line placement can also find themselves in the same scenario, but instead focused on PICC line placement and solely on the outcomes of PICC lines alone. A dedicated PICC team does have clinicians who are full time in the placement and care of PICC lines, but oftentimes vascular access devices outside of the PICC line take a secondary level. A new generation of vascular access has grown out of the combination of the traditional IV team and dedicated PICC team, which is more encompassing. This type of approach has been termed the vascular access service. In essence the word team implies more than one individual, so it may be the facility can only afford one clinician who becomes a proceduralist, placing only PICC lines and that is their entire function or they can justify the hiring of multiple clinicians who can move from just the placement of a PICC line into adding additional functions from the vascular access continuum of care and not just become a technical PICC line inserter.

15.3   Creation of the PICC Team

Teams specializing in vascular access have been created by various departments or managers in the healthcare arena. In the late 1990s, with the advent of homecare in the United States, PICC line usage increased, especially in light of the AIDS crisis. A change in reimbursement for homecare with a fixed case rate resulted in the elimination of payment for the placement of a PICC line in the homecare arena. In order to discharge a patient without enduring increased length of stays, hospitals in the United States had to initiate PICC line insertion programs. The patient had to have a PICC line in place on discharge or alternate infusion would not accept the patient. As a result, PICC lines were placed by nurses, interventional radiologists, technicians, or surgeons. With the tightening of reimbursement structures, PICC line placement was established via the PICC team, IV team, or vascular access specialty for placement, with interventional radiology taking a backseat to placements. PICC line insertion programs are initiated by various departments in a facility. Implementation of PICC line insertion program may start with the creation of one lone clinician who covers the entire inpatient and outpatient arena or may be an add-on procedure to an existing IV team or physician service.

- As noted by Burns [11] and Burns and Lamberth [12], the Interventional Radiology Department can become overwhelmed with PICC line orders that involve a low-skill procedure with minimal reimbursement. In order to reduce patient delay, a nurse or technician team was started out of the Radiology Department. These teams may become only device inserters in a procedural room as noted by Burns and Lamberth [12] or may blossom as Burns [11] points out into a full vascular access service, with multiple full-time clinicians, as in the case of Vanderbilt University Medical Center. Burns [11] notes that the team growth included the addition of acute care central venous catheter insertions (CVCs), as well as the implementation of a pediatric PICC line program.
- Carroll and Lashbrook [14] note that Bronson Methodist Hospital's team was established early on by a physician in the 1990s, with the sole purpose of reducing infections associated with the administration of total parenteral nutrition (TPN). This team, which initiated PICC line placements on TPN patients, evolved into a team of 10 nurses, who place lines, manage lines, educate staff, and perform vascular access assessment. Their original goal to reduce infection

has now resulted in recognition for an almost zero infection rate for 7 years while placing over 1,000 PICC lines a year.

- Ean et al. [19] at Mayo Clinic cites the initiation of the PICC program from the Department of Nursing. A traditional IV team or service was currently part of the Mayo Clinic nursing program design. PICC line placement was added to the responsibilities of the existing IV team as PICC lines were ordered for discharge to alternate sites. PICC lines became a necessary vascular access device for inpatients and outpatients leaving the facility. MD Anderson Cancer Center's PICC team was also birthed from the traditional IV team as well.

- Horsby et al. [23] cited that the program at Covenant Medical Center was started out of nursing to provide a reliable vascular access device for inpatients, as well as provide a reliable device for outpatients. This facility has created an outpatient PICC line placement service that advertises to local alternate site care, physician offices, and other local hospitals. The increase in outpatient procedures, which are reimbursed a procedural fee unlike inpatients, which are based on an all inclusive fee, has resulted in providing a revenue stream to the service.

- Sir Run Run Shaw Hospital in China, which is a partner hospital of Loma Linda University Hospital in California, initiated a PICC line team out of the oncology service, for chemotherapeutic drug delivery in patient's. The PICC line team expanded from a departmental service focused on oncology PICC lines to an entire hospital service focused on vascular access assessment and PICC line placement. This is the first hospital to place a triple-lumen PICC line in the critical care setting in China with the champion being Zhao Linfang the PICC team director. The team implemented an early assessment program with an algorithm approved by the physician staff in 2012.

- Santollim et al. [34] cites that the PICC line placement service was initiated out of the specialty of orthopedics, with a focus on infections and antibiotic delivery. The Institute of Orthopedics and Traumatology of Hospital das Clinicas de Faculdade de Medicina da Universidade de Sao Paulo, Brazil, initiated the program with one initial PICC line placer and has grown into a team approach within the facility. This team implements an early assessment process with an algorithm in 2010. Nursing team members were given the autonomy to select the appropriate vascular access device for the patient, whether that be a PIV, PICC, tunneled catheter, or port. What started as a lone PICC placer has grown into a process, which has demonstrated a decrease in phlebitis, reduction of multiple cannulations, reduced patient pain, and improved patient satisfaction.

- Dobson et al. [17] discusses the creation of a PICC team at Banner Estrella Medical Center. As the nursing team inserting PICC lines was an as-needed team, it became evident that a full-time dedicated process was necessary. The respiratory therapy department showed an interest in taking over the service full time and incorporated the job function into their existing duties. The respiratory team moved forward into the placement of acute care CVCs and ultrasound-guided PIVs. The respiratory therapy team was already placing arterial catheters.

- Alexandrou et al. [2] initiated a program at a university hospital in Southwest Sydney placing acute care CVCs. The initiation of the program was to reduce the workload on physicians and residents, as well as provide improved outcomes, with a limited highly trained dedicated staff of nurses performing the procedure repetitively. PICC line placement was adopted into this already existing service out of the ICU (intensive care unit). This program was initiated in 1996.

The PICC line team or service can be formulated out of multiple areas of the hospital from ICU, nursing service, existing IV team, specialty service such as orthopedics or oncology, interventional radiology, and nutritional support to respiratory therapy. In the literature PICC line teams have been created out of almost any department in the healthcare setting. The key to the development of a PICC line team is a champion and patient need.

15.4 Champion and Rationale for the Creation of a PICC Team

A champion is the basis for the creation of any new process. A champion is an individual who supports and speaks up for a cause [27]. Champions recognize the need to improve a situation or remedy problems. The champion to create a PICC line team varies from facility to facility. As noted above, the PICC line team is not necessarily created by the same department or title. Who is the champion for the creation of a PICC team [2, 10–12, 14, 17–19, 23, 25, 29, 34]?

- Physicians who have a vested interest in improving patient safety, reducing infections, reducing complications, and improving patient satisfaction. Especially by the fact that the majority of PICC lines are now placed with ultrasound and soon to be ECG, insertion complications and patient flow are greatly improved.
- Radiology or operating room that wants to open procedural areas and improve patient flow as well as improve reimbursement by using high-tech suites for higher-tech procedures.
- Intensive care unit that wants to improve the timeliness of insertions and reduce delays in therapy especially in light of the sepsis protocols or bundles.
- Nursing department heads that want to improve outcomes from complications such as phlebitis, infiltration, and extravasation. Oftentimes a nursing manager from patient quality, patient safety, or patient satisfaction will prompt the development of a PICC team.
- Pharmacy department that wants to facilitate medication delivery in a timely manner and not endure costly drug wastage.
- Infection control or an infectious disease physician that wants to have a dedicated highly trained staff to place central lines, thereby reducing central line insertion infections and potentially care infections.
- Case managers or care managers have prompted the development of a PICC team to facilitate decreased length of stay by enabling the patient to receive mid- to long-term care in an ambulatory setting or homecare.
- Specialty departments such as neonatal ICU, pediatrics, oncology, and orthopedics create PICC teams in order to facilitate infusion delivery for mid- to long-term patients or reduce the complications of multiple venipunctures, phlebitis, and infiltrations from harsh infusates.

In the published literature, the rationale for the creation of a PICC line team is almost the same from article to article. The main reasons are cited below [2, 6, 10–12, 14, 17, 18, 23, 25, 29, 34, 35]:

- Improvement of patient outcomes
  - Reduced phlebitis, infiltration, and extravasation
  - Reduced pneumothorax, arterial puncture, and air embolism
  - Reduced insertion and post insertion-related infections
  - Reduction of multiple venipunctures
  - Improvement in patient assessment for the proper vascular access device
  - Safety for patients who are not candidates for a CVAD placed in the jugular or subclavian vein
  - Alternative to the femoral CVAD which is prone to high infection rates
- Improvement of patient experience or satisfaction
  - Reduced needlesticks
  - Improved and timely medication delivery
  - Timely service without lengthy wait time
- Improvement of patient flow
  - Reduction of bottlenecks to getting placement
  - Timely insertion for critical areas such as ICU
  - Timely patient discharge and reduction of length of stays
  - Facilitate blood draws
  - Oncology patients who have power injectable procedures
- Improvement of cost efficiencies
  - Reduction in complication treatment from phlebitis, infiltration, infection, extravasation, pneumothorax, and arterial puncture
  - Reduction in drug wastage and timely delivery of medications
  - Reduction in material supplies and labor for repeated PIV insertions
  - Implementation of early vascular access assessment at admission to reduce repeated procedures

A PICC line is no longer the hidden vascular access device but one that is widely used worldwide. The rationale behind its use is reliable infusate delivery with very low complications. If one were to look at the two major complications of symptomatic treatable thrombosis and infection and lump them together, it would not result in more than 5 % [14, 22] of the population who receives a PICC line. Ultrasound guidance has improved outcomes significantly over the last decade as well as the infection control bundle. Ninety-five percent of patients experience no major complications. For patients who have limited venous access or are receiving infusate therapy that is irritating or have vesicant potential, the PICC line has proved to be a valuable tool in the catheter selection categories.

15.5 Duties of the PICC Team or a Vascular Access Service

Infusion therapy is more complex, and virtually every patient in a care setting is now receiving some type of infusion therapy. This therapy may be short term, long term, or provided in various settings of the hospital, ambulatory care, homecare, skilled care nursing facility, or nursing home. Determining the best vascular access device to complete the patient's therapy with the best outcomes has become the strategic goal. Technology associated with the placement of vascular access devices and their care has expanded over the last decade. As in the United States alone, there are over 300 million PIVs (peripheral intravenous catheters) sold as well as over 7 million central venous catheters [21]. This does not include the arterial, intraosseous, subcutaneous, and intraspinal procedures performed per year. Knowledge of the clinician has become critical in the vascular access space, besides the procedural competency [21]. The labor demands to place devices, care for devices, troubleshoot devices, monitor outcomes, and assess patients have become overwhelming. It is now a house-wide initiative, as facilities cannot hire enough full-time staff to implement every aspect of the vascular access continuum of care. Vascular access is multidisciplinary involving pharmacists, physicians, care coordinators, clinicians, infection prevention, and quality, patient safety, and patient satisfaction departments of the facility. Having a dedicated vascular access service becomes the foundation of this continuum, to facilitate the integration of all aspects of this multidisciplinary approach.

Published literature identifies the duties and functions of a vascular access service, PICC team, and IV team. These teams may be composed of nurses, respiratory therapists, advanced nurse practitioners, physician assistants, and physicians. A composite of those duties is presented below for consideration when creating a team or process [1, 11, 14, 23, 25, 28, 32, 34, 35]:

- Creation of a vascular access assessment process, tool, algorithm, and decision tree with a multidisciplinary team of pharmacists, physicians, and clinicians vested in vascular access. To be followed by the creation of an educational program on vascular access assessment for all clinicians and physicians in the facility
- Vascular access placement or the assisting of the placement of (PICC lines, midlines, PIVs, central venous catheters, dialysis catheters, ports, and tunneled catheters) with ultrasound guidance, modified Seldinger®, Seldinger® technique, tip navigation, and tip location (ECG)
- Provide troubleshooting advice and training to clinical staff
- Data collection and reporting (outcome monitoring and patient satisfaction)
- Infusion product evaluation and implementation
- Investigation (root cause analysis) of infections and adverse events related to vascular access
- Development of:
  - Policies and procedures (vascular access placement, insertion complication management, post insertion complication management, device selection, care and maintenance, and removal)
  - Patient educational materials and development of patient consent process
  - Clinical staff training competencies
  - Outcome monitoring tools
- Implementation of:
  - Infection prevention program for vascular access device infections (CR-BSI or CLA-BSI) with compliance monitoring
  - Program to reduce needlesticks and blood exposure to staff members

- Involvement in:
  - Sepsis bundle
  - Rapid response team
  - Infection prevention committee
  - Rounding on device necessity and reduction of femoral lines
- Performance or competency training of staff on:
  - Dressing changes
  - Accessory device changes
  - Flushing
  - Placement of PIVs
  - Blood draws from line or peripherally
  - Port access and deaccess
  - Device removal
  - Blood draws for cultures
  - Total parenteral nutrition administration

The duties of a true vascular access service are labor intensive and not all facilities might be able to accomplish a true version of this program. At that point, the facility must question what their needs are. Is it competency and skill in device placement alone? If that is the case, a procedural team placing specific vascular access devices with a high level of competency might be the financial alternative. Education and competency training on care and maintenance and troubleshooting might have to be provided by an alternative department, in the facility. Outcome monitoring although the basis for performance improvement might have to be forgone or provided by staff, from quality or infection prevention. This leads to the key initiative, which is patient assessment for the most appropriate vascular access device to meet the therapy and patients needs. Barton and Danek [7] defined the desired state for vascular access as follows: "on admission, the patient will have a vascular access plan that meets his/her needs. The plan will be re-evaluated at regular intervals or as the patient condition changes." In order to accomplish such a goal, clinical staff would have to be educated on a process that is created by a multidisciplinary team. It is difficult to create a process without the vested interest of a vascular access team of some origin. A team only dedicated to competency in vascular access placement runs the risk of not being able to implement a comprehensive vascular access assessment program for device planning.

Bolton [10] discusses a business case for the expansion of a traditional IV therapy team. In 1998, the IV team's main role was to place PIVs, author and implement policies, educate staff on IV therapy, and audit services within the trust. In 2001, the team added a nurse-led PICC insertion service. Initially the PICC service provided for a limited number of specialties such as oncology, TPN patients, and respiratory patients requiring antibiotics. As the demands for PICC line insertion increased, the rate of PIV phlebitis and staff adherence to policy declined. The IV team had changed from educating and advising to a PICC line insertion service. An additional six full-time nurses were added to the team to allow for time to perform PIVs, educate staff, implement care bundles, and insert PICC lines. Staffing is critical to the development of a program consisting of competency in insertion, planning, monitoring, and educating ancillary staff. A business case may need to be developed to add additional staffing to proceed beyond the skilled placement of PICC lines with dedicated full-time labor hours.

15.6   Training on the Placement of a PICC Line (Didactic)

Choosing and training a clinician to place a PICC line or become a vascular access specialist is the foundation to a successful program. The individual or group of individuals provides the framework and backbone of a program. Programs have failed on the basis of the skill, knowledge, and motivation of the individual hired. The individual chosen must have the passion to start a new initiative and the patience to learn a skill.

Vascular access specialists or PICC line placers should have the following characteristics or traits:

Self-starters and entrepreneurial
Analytical and out-of-the-box thinkers with well-developed critical thinking skills
Not afraid to try new things
Good hand–eye coordination
Work well independently and in teams
Comfortable with scalpels, wires, and introducers
Good communication skills with doctors, patients, and staff
Critical care and emergency room backgrounds might be a plus
Knowledge of sterile technique and skill in placing PIVs

In addition to finding and hiring the right clinician, it is important to train this clinician. Moureau et al. [30] recommend utilizing a training logbook as a checklist to verify completion of all the training steps of the training process. If the trainee fails to pass a step, he/she has to repeat the performance until able to demonstrate competence. An international evidence-based consensus task force was established through the World Congress of Vascular Access (WoCoVA) to provide definitions and recommendations for training and insertion of CVADs (central venous access devices). Training consists of a didactic, practicum, testing process, and proctorship. The panel of experts recommends the following topics be covered during the didactic section of an educational course on CVADs. The Consensus Task Force recommends a 6–8-h didactic education as a time element [30]:

- Didactic course
  - Anatomy and physiology of relevant body systems
    - Venous and arterial anatomy of the arms, axillary, neck, and chest
    - Peripheral nerve identification and distribution
    - Blood flow dynamics and Virchow's triad
    - Respiratory and cardiac systems as applicable
  - Ultrasound for insertion and assessment
    - Image optimization and analysis
    - Vessel size and patency
    - Knobology and probe types

- Central venous device tip location
  - Tip verification (x-ray, ECG, Doppler, and navigation basics)
  - Tip location (at or near the cavo-atrial junction)
- Infection control and sterile technique
  - Hand washing, maximal sterile barrier, and skin antisepsis
  - Use of carts or kits with all components for the procedure
  - Empowerment to stop the procedure and checklists
  - Evaluation of device necessity
- Device selection and indications
  - Patient assessment (infusates, length of therapy, labs, medical history)
  - Catheter materials and composition
  - Size and features (flow, power injection, gauge, lumens)
  - Indications and contraindications for PICC line placement
- Insertion procedures, complication prevention, evaluation, and management
  - Landmark and ultrasound techniques
  - Introduction methods (Peel-Away sheath, modified Seldinger® technique, and Seldinger® technique for fluoroscopy
  - Use of local anesthetics
- Care and maintenance
  - Dressing changes, securement devices, flushing protocols, connector disinfection, and thrombolytic management
- Legal, patient consents and outcome monitoring, qualification, and competency
- Neonates and children (if applicable)
  - Insertion with and without ultrasound or near-infrared technology
  - Anatomy and physiology specific to the population
  - Insertion and post insertion complications specific to the population
  - Use of anesthetics specific to the population

15.7 Training on the Placement of a PICC Line (Practicum and Testing)

Following the didactic, it is recommended that the learner proceeds to the next training step the practicum or simulated practice. Completion of a course does not indicate competency to perform the procedure, and oftentimes the attendance of a course is misconstrued as the attendee is a "PICC-certified clinician." Completion of the course signifies the clinician merely attended a PICC line instruction course but does not have the skills at this point to place a PICC line independently with competency. The course must be followed up with a simulation laboratory and proctorship on live patient insertions, which is overseen by a skilled practitioner in PICC line placement. The WoCoVA Consensus Task Force suggests a 4-h hands-on training on inanimate models and in addition suggests a 6-h hands-on training on normal human volunteers, for detection of normal ultrasound anatomy [30].

The practicum consists of:

- Anatomical model simulation for placement and measuring
- Model simulation for ultrasound basics

There are a variety of inanimate models that are used for practicums to simulate the placement procedure steps, as well as to simulate the venous anatomy. Procedurally there is the Peter PICC LineTM simulator, which contains the basilic, cephalic, median basilic, jugular, and subclavian veins, as well as palpable ribs. The simulator allows the placer to practice sterile technique, palpation of veins, measurement techniques, catheter introduction, and catheter threading. For ultrasound simulation, the Blue Phantom is available. The Blue Phantom IV arm allows one to practice their ultrasound training skills by utilizing simulated human tissue. This simulator allows the clinician to practice ultrasound system controls, transducer positioning and movement, recognition of the venous anatomy, and using ultrasound to target the appropriate vessel for cannulation. Additionally low-cost inanimate models such as turkey breasts have been used for simulation practice with ultrasound [30]. A low-cost alternative is to use human volunteers for scanning and measuring techniques [30]. Human volunteers however are not useful to practice insertion techniques which leave the Peter PICC Line™ as the target simulator for simulated insertion. The Infusion Nursing Standards of Practice [24] discourages the performance of invasive procedures on peers due to health risks for the peer-volunteer; however, noninvasive scanning is completely acceptable.

Educational competency usually results in a testing mechanism of some type. Testing can be oral, written on-site, or written on line via a web-based course. At this point in time, not all PICC line training programs encompass some type of testing mechanism. On-site courses oftentimes provide a certificate of attendance at the end of the didactic course with or without practicum. This certificate does not indicate the attendee is competent but rather that they attended the curriculum. The WoCoVA Consensus Task Force [30] contends that a trainee must be able to demonstrate educational competence with a testing mechanism. They state the educational competence should be evaluated with a multiple-choice test of at least 100 questions. The trainee must then pass with at least 70 % correct answers before proceeding to the hands-on training exam. The hands-on audit assesses the practical skills acquired during the training process. The trainee must pass the entire practical steps before continuing to live proctored insertions on patients in the healthcare environment. As stated, not all educational programs have a written or practicum training testing protocol measurement for competency. This is a new recommendation made by the WoCoVA Consensus Task Force in 2013 [30]. Testing provides some methodology to ascertain knowledge and competency and should be highly considered in training programs.

15.8 Training on the Placement of a PICC Line (Proctoring and Competency)

The final step to complete a training program is usually proctored supervised insertions on patients in the facility. Supervised procedures are a critical step in ascertaining the competency of a clinician to perform the procedure in a safe manner. The number of supervised procedures has not been firmly established in the literature. The Infusion Nursing Standards of Practice [24] suggests that the employer or facility maintains a written policy and procedure for PICC line insertion that establishes the requirements for competency and supervision and that this documentation is in the employee's records. Of note, the Consensus Task Force from WoCoVA did conclude that the supervisors who are proctoring and training must have full competence in device placement and must maintain their skills through their clinical activity.

A literature search into the number of proctored and simulated procedures for competency was undertaken. Publications obtained offered the following advice to the number of proctored insertions:

- Sznajder et al. [36] suggests that operator training and experiences are critical. The article goes on to state that clinicians who have placed more than 50 central venous catheters have less than half the complication rates of clinicians who have less than 50 catheterization attempts. Do 50 insertions have to be proctored, or at 50 insertions, does the skill set become finely tuned?

- The American College of Chest Physicians (United States 1998) [5] determines that the competency learning curve for central venous catheterization is 10–20 procedures without ultrasound.

- Davis and Kokotis [16] suggested that three observations of successful insertions and three proctored insertions, as being the basis for placing independently. The addition of a trainee observing the placement of a PICC line by a skilled practitioner might provide reinforcement in the steps to performing the procedure.

- The Royal College of Radiologists (United Kingdom 2005) [15] places the competency number at 25 vascular line insertions. The organization also states that different trainees will acquire the skill at different rates, so the end point should be assessed by the individual learner.

- Petit and Wycoff [31], in the National Association of Neonatal Nurses (NANN/United States) PICC Guidelines, suggest that three proctored successful insertions of a PICC line are required prior to placing independently.

- Kopman [26] personally concludes that five to ten proctored insertions might be advised for competency validation in the placement of central venous catheters.

- The American College of Emergency Physicians (United States 2008) [5] recommends 25 documented and reviewed cases with ultrasound, for a new learner placing central venous access catheters.

- Ramirez et al. [33] suggests that five proctored successful insertions in the placement of an internal jugular central venous catheter are necessary prior to independent placements.

- Breschan et al. [9] suggest that in neonates weighing less than 4.5 kg, around 15 cannulations are needed to be comfortable with the placement of central vascular access devices.

- The American Board of Internal Medicine (United States 2013) [4] does not specify a minimum number of procedures to demonstrate competency in central venous access placement but states the clinician should have adequate knowledge and understanding of the procedures and each resident should be an active participant for each procedure five or more times.

The bottom line is that competency for placement of a vascular access device ranges from three observed with three successful placements to a maximum of 50 insertions pre-ultrasound. It is clear that there is no magic number for observations or proctored placements and that each institution should determine within their own facility what deems one qualified or competent to perform a procedure independently. The methodology of see one, do one, and teach one is no longer a valid teaching process in the placement of any vascular access device. The Consensus Task force (WoCoVA) [30] has suggested utilizing a global rating scale and checklist. The task force contends that the placement of a central venous access device (CVAD) is predictable; therefore, the assessment of the procedure can be performed using a checklist, with each step or skill mapped out. Utilizing a minimum or maximum number of procedures for competency evaluation does not account for the various learning curves of each individual. As previously mentioned, some clinicians are apt to master the procedure faster than other clinicians and vice versa.

This brings up the question of how many procedures per month or year equate to maintaining procedural competency and how many procedures should be reviewed per year by a proctor to ascertain competency has been consistent. Is the placement of one PICC line a month or 12 PICC lines per year enough to maintain competency and more importantly sterile technique? In choosing a facility or doctor as a patient, would I as the author choose a facility or doctor who performs a procedure once a month? The placement of a vascular access device has evolved over the last decade with changes in technological advancement and infection prevention strategies. What is the minimum number of procedures performed yearly to adhere to guideline changes or utilize new technology? The number is actually unknown. Anecdotally it has been suggested that the placement of 200 central venous access devices per year is likely to enable the user to adopt new technology and adhere to guideline changes. This number is based on Bass and Bashore [8] who suggested that a minimum of 200 or more coronary arterial interventional procedures be performed per year in the hospital setting by a physician to ascertain yearly minimal competency. This article has been highly debated in the medical arena, as requiring too many procedures per year. In the model of training clinicians in units all over the facility to place PICC lines, Hornsby et al. [23] coined the phrase "PICC, Stick, and Run Teams." In this scenario, it was costly to continue to provide training and retraining. The end result of this cycle was not the development of a competent team but the exercise of continuous training and proctoring. The economics of the situation has to be taken into consideration. Is it less costly to have fewer inserters who place a higher number of devices or multiple inserters who place fewer devices? The issue related to the number of insertions per year to maintain competency might be resolved with economics and the cost of training versus justifying a minimum number of procedures per year. The question is: how many clinicians in a facility can you keep abreast of guideline and technological changes?

15.9 Economics

Worldwide healthcare costs are rising and under scrutiny. It would be no surprise that a team placing vascular access devices, maintaining those devices, and providing education would be considered a luxury. The real question is a dedicated team or service a luxury or does it provide cost savings to the facility in labor, materials, reduced complications, reduced liability, and length of patient stay.

A nursing study by Barton and Danek [7] at the University of Florida exemplifies the implementation of a proactive approach to vascular access planning at admission for the patient and the subsequent length of stay cost savings. The study findings indicate that 22,589 patients received infusion therapy in 1995 and that 25 % of these patients had infusion therapy for 7 or more days. This means peripheral infusion therapy was used exclusively for 5,756 patients who had therapy for 7 or more days. A little over half of those patients received a central line or midline, but 2,878 patients who had 7 days or more of infusate therapy had multiple PIV cannulations. In essence, 13 % of the patients had only a PIV and had infusion therapy for over 7 days. This prompted a 4-week prospective review of 371 patients. The review indicated that the average number of attempts for a successful PIV cannulation was 2.18 with a range of 1–14 attempts. In addition, 27 % of the patients had a treatment delay, as a result of IV complications or lack of available access. To provide reliable infusate delivery, the hospital implemented a vascular access planning algorithm with physician and clinical education. The results published in the hospital newsletter subsequent to their article indicate that a reduction of length of hospital stay occurred by 2 days and the projected savings was $500,000 (USA) per year. The authors stated that good decision making regarding the type of vascular access device at the onset of therapy helps to improve the overall patient's satisfaction, avoiding delays of therapy, and reduce length of stay.

Bolton [10] at a UK hospital discovered that when the IV team begun to place PICC lines, a shortage of labor occurred. As a result, PIV complication rates for phlebitis and infection increased. A business case was developed to demonstrate the increased costs of treating complications versus the addition of six additional full-time employees to the IV team to handle the increased usage of PICC lines, provide staffing education, and assess PIV sites for complications or alternative devices. Upon approval, the implementation resulted in a net cash savings of $170,000 (pounds) in labor, materials, and complication reduction. The main premise being that if cannulae are inserted by inexperienced staff, the risk of trauma and infection increases. In this case study, PICC line usage increased from 245 (2006) to 501 (2007). It is likely that vascular access planning became part of the labor change, although it is not cited. What is cited is that in 2007, 1,611 staff members were educated in a classroom setting and 1,487 patients were seen by the IV team/PICC team.

Economically the placement of a PICC line, in the Interventional Radiology Department (IR) or operating room (OR), results in a very high-cost procedure with high operational cost losses in labor (3 staff members) and materials, as well as making this high-tech suite unavailable for procedures, involving a higher reimbursement or technical skill. The interruption of patient flow to take a patient from the unit to the high-tech procedure room and back interrupts productivity and likely delays patient care. If the schedule is full, the PICC line placement is often shifted 1 or 2 days at an additional cost in length of stay for the facility. Hornsby et al. [23] cite the cost of placement of a PICC line in the IR at $450–$3,000 (USA) and the cost at bedside to range from $150 to $200 (USA). PICC lines placed in this setting often require the utilization of fluoroscopy which is an unnecessary radiation exposure for the patient, as well as a cost loss to the facility. The cost savings with a point of service shift of PICC line placement from the IR to the patient bedside with nursing were estimated at $300 to $2,800 per procedure. Hornsby et al. [23] cite that the hospital realized a savings of up to $175,200 a year by shifting the PICC lines out of the IR procedure rooms. Bedside insertion success in cannulation for PICC lines placed by a dedicated full-time PICC team was at 93–95 %. Additional authors cited savings by shifting PICC lines from IR and OR to nursing. Santolucito [36] quoted a savings of $383,000 (USA) a year and Dobson and Wong [17] cited a savings of $125,273 (USA) a year. Economically the cost of utilizing a high-cost procedure room designed for an emergent or higher acuity procedure is not economically sound for the hospital management. This is especially true if the hospital operates on a fixed reimbursement rate or structured yearly operational budget. It has been noted that a PICC line procedure ties up a suite for approximately 1 h although the physician may only be in the procedure for 10–15 min. The room turn time includes patient transfer, setup, and cleanup, all of which do not involve the physicians time.

In international countries the short-term acute care central venous catheter (CVC) has been traditionally utilized for vascular access in oncology and mid- to long-term infectious disease treatment. The acute care CVC is placed as well upon venous exhaustion from multiple PIVs that have encountered infiltration, phlebitis, patient pullout, and extravasation. The cost of the CVC itself remains low; however, the cost of additional materials for placement in the form of maximal sterile barrier precautions has raised the operational cost. Labor is another cost as there are likely one or two assistants to assist in the placement procedure. In some situations, the patient is taken to the OR suite for placement, which adds a higher procedural cost to the placement. As the CVC is perceived as a low-cost vascular access central line, it has become the go-to VAD. "Is the CVC indeed low cost?" becomes the question. If the CVC is placed in an expensive OR suite, the operational cost is likely to have increased tenfold. If a patient gets a new CVC on each admission for chemotherapy involving a 3–6-month cycle, the insertion cost for a PICC line is likely equivalent to the cost of multiple CVCs, as the PICC line remains in place for the length of treatment as a long-term VAD. The concern with CVCs is also one of complications. Complications and their treatment are not a low-cost expenditure. The Agency for Healthcare Research and Quality [3] in the United States has cited the cost of a pneumothorax at $17,000–$45,000 [3] (USA) with an additional length of hospital stay at 4–7 days. Litigation costs in the United States are a prime concern, and the American Society of Anesthesiology Closed Claims Project (1996) cites the average litigation settlement for pneumothorax at $143,250 [20]. CVC placement can involve complications not associated with PICC line placement such as pneumothorax, major arterial puncture, air embolism, and vessel perforation. In addition, the risk of sending a patient to an alternate setting with an acute care catheter can potentially result in air embolism and patient bleed out. Removal of an acute care CVC carries a higher risk of air embolism if not performed properly, as well as dressed properly. Current literature does not compare the costs of complications for a PICC versus a CVC but has up to this point compared the purchase cost of a PICC to the purchase cost of an acute CVC. There is more to cost effectiveness besides material acquisition costs. The decision to utilize the most appropriate device for the patient's safety, medical condition, and length of treatment needs to be considered. Patients may not want to leave the facility with an acute CVC versus a PICC line from a perceived comfort and satisfaction level.

15.10 Productivity

Time and motion are the basis for staffing a PICC team, and it is imperative that the time to perform a variety of tasks is monitored and collected. Without this data, it becomes difficult to increase the number of full-time employees or part-time employee additions to the team. Working short staff decreases the satisfaction of not only the employee, but the entire continuum of care is impacted. The lack of labor hour resources can result in a delay of therapy, increased patient complications, longer length of patient stays, wastage of infusates, overtime hours, and employee turnover.

Burns [11] stated that the team must establish a clear scheduling process for PICC line orders and a system by which the orders are transmitted to the team in a just-in-time process. The team as Burns [11] states then determines the placement queue of the order, based on the triage of patent needs. With the evolution of electronic medical records, orders are often transmitted electronically, but some facilities may still need to work on the basis of phone orders, fax orders, or pager orders.

Service hours provided by PICC teams vary; however, the optimal system is one that performs the duties of a vascular access service 24 h a day and 7 days a week. One of the prime rationales is to take an active part in the rapid response process of sepsis identification. Some facilities have mandated central line placement within 30 min to 4 h as part of their internal sepsis bundle. The PICC line has become an integral part of the sepsis bundle. Depending on labor available, teams may have to choose to staff limited hours of just 5–7 days a week on the day shift or they may choose to stagger employees to try to cover a 10–12-h time period. Today's medicine is a 24-h business proposition and the patient is in need of reliable access 24 h a day. Providing service for a partial day does potentially cause a delay of therapy and possibly discharge. Teams that are understaffed will find themselves shifting critical line placements to the next day, leaving the patient with alternative vascular access that might not have been the best assessment choice. Some teams will provide an afterhours service on-call or an outside contractor will fill in for holidays, weekends, and nights.

Care technicians have been incorporated into the PICC line teams in many facilities. These technicians are low-cost assistants to the clinician placing PICC lines. The care technician can assist in gathering supplies, cleaning up after procedures, assisting with supplies during the procedure, and observing and filling out the checklist for sterile technique. A care technician can be empowered to stop a procedure for a break in sterile technique and provides a second set of eyes to the sterile field, as well as becoming the traffic cop, stopping those who would enter the room during the procedure [11].

Productivity includes the capturing of time and motion data. An internal study should be conducted to determine the amount of time it takes to perform a procedure, troubleshoot a problem, educate clinical staff and patients, monitor and analyze outcomes, as well as take part in collaborative meetings within the department and external to the department. When conducting time audits, it is crucial to determine the time elements of the entire procedure. For instance, procedure time is not just the time to insert a device but the time to walk to the room, review the chart, meet with the clinical caregiver, collect supplies, wash hands, initiate and finish the procedure, clean up post procedure, and documentation. In some instances, there may be follow-up time in addition to the procedure such as reviewing x-rays, consulting with another specialist to place an unsuccessful attempt, logging outcomes into an internal database, transmitting information to an alternate service provider or physician, and managing a malposition or another insertion complication. Often clinicians think only of the procedure itself and not the entire process. It is surprising how often a patient has to use the restroom right before the procedure and the PICC line inserter is performing the task of assisting the patient to the restroom. Alexander [1] cites the time to place a PIV at 15 min; however, Terry et al. [37] cites the time to place a difficult PIV at 40 min with more than one attempt. It is critical to identify by time the easy patients from the difficult patients, as the difficult patient will steal away labor hours that are necessary to the functioning of a team. One of the key elements in determining the time element for a procedure is not to present an inaccurate picture. Often clinicians are so enamored with presenting how fast they can do a procedure without really understanding what time element they are committing themselves to. The author often asks clinicians how long it takes to place a PIV. The routine answer is 5 min. If it does take 5 min from start to finish to place a PIV, then a clinician from an IV team can place two PIVs every 10 min and 12-h or almost 100 in an 8-h day. This is not even realistic when one imagines walking to the patients room, having a conversation with the patient and clinical staff, performing the most difficult insertions which sometimes require ultrasound, and maintaining a no-touch or sterile technique. It is very important to set a realistic time and motion goal and to staff accordingly.

The time to place a PICC line varies by setting, amount of staffing in the procedure room, patient ease or difficulty, and organizational process. Terry et al. [37] cites the time to place a PICC line at 120 min, and Alexander et al. [1] cites the time at 90 min. Does that 30 min differential matter? Since 2005, the PICC line insertion has involved maximal sterile barrier precautions. What impact to the time element has the addition of steps to the procedure added? Has the procedure changed allowing for a savings of 30 min due to new technology or has the procedure time actually increased as a result of infection prevention and tip location and tip navigation? Meyer [28] provides a table of sample productivity numbers, as well how to calculate productivity. It is imperative that the team creates their own numbers based on their own facility, process, techniques, and tools. All systems are not created equal and the patient flow may differ greatly from facility to facility. Time will once again vary if the patient is coming to a procedure room or the clinician is performing the procedure at bedside. Even if the patient is coming to a procedure room, one must account for the time of the transporter or the check-in process for an outpatient. All of these factors are part of the overall time to place a PICC line. It may not represent clinical procedural time but it does represent facility productivity time. A good suggestion is to take each function and break down the time to perform each element of that function. This will enable you to get an accurate time representation. For instance, various time elements are involved in the placement of a PICC line with some sample elements listed below:

- Transport time
- Entire procedural time (includes arriving at the room to documentation of the procedure)
- X-ray time (ordering, taking, and obtaining x-ray results (if ECG is not utilized))
- Malposition correction time

Time and motion must be evaluated from the perspective of an individual acting alone or in a team of two. For instance, an individual acting alone may take 90–120 min to perform a PICC line insertion from start to finish; however, an individual acting in a team of two would have double the labor and be able to complete the procedure in possibly half the time. With the advent of additional infection precautions and the reduction of malpositions with tip navigation and the reduction of x-rays with tip location, the time element to the placement of a PICC line has likely increased on the PICC inserters' part. On the back side, however, the time saved in not correcting malpositions and not waiting for an x-ray or reviewing an x-ray has shortened the time in other aspects of the patient flow process. Time must be reviewed from a broader perspective and complete picture and not just procedural time.

If the time to place a PICC line from start to finish with correction, and line release is 90 min for a practitioner acting alone, then in an 8-h day it is feasible that a clinician may perform 6 PICC lines per day. However, if the time element is 120 min, then a clinician may perform 4 PICC lines in an 8-h day. When reviewing those numbers, one must realize that this clinician is only performing PICC line insertions and does not have the time element to handle dressing changes, troubleshooting, declotting, and education. In this case scenario, the PICC placer is just a placer and is only concerned with the line on insertion and not post insertion. The clinician can place 20–30 PICC lines a week in an 8-h day or 900–1,350 PICC lines in 45 workweeks. Forty-five workweeks are utilized to account for vacation and holidays. Is this the actual number that a clinician can really place per year? Undoubtedly, the PICC team of one or more clinicians will be called to perform difficult sticks, provide education, troubleshoot, declot lines, measure outcomes, participate in committees, author policies and procedures, or become the go-to person for every vascular access issue or question in the facility. One cannot plan a team of one or more individuals based only on insertions but must build a buffer of time element to encompass the vascular access picture. Inevitably the one person who places PICC lines becomes the go-to person for all other aspects of vascular access necessitating an increase in full-time employees (FTEs). One becomes the start of an actual team with a shared goal of vascular access patient outcomes related to their performance and functions. The author in 2005 [25] cited that one FTE is approximately 800 PICC line placements per year with the intention of providing a buffer for growth and that this individual would become the vascular access resource in the facility. The Field of Dreams movie quoted that "if you build it, they will come," and it remains true that if you build the first FTE in PICC line placement, it will begin to gravitate towards becoming a team, encompassing a broader picture in the institution in providing vascular access. Productivity and time and motion are paramount to the successful implementation of a PICC team. This topic alone would likely represent a chapter.

Conclusion

A PICC team is not necessarily a lone PICC line placer in the facility, as that is likely a proceduralist. A PICC team is also not likely the training of nurses throughout the institution to place PICC lines in their spare time, as they do not necessarily work towards a common outcome goal in synergy. A PICC team is likely to have multiple members and may perform multiple tasks that include care and maintenance as well as troubleshooting and clinical staff education. Two components not yet discussed due to time element are outcomes monitoring and the implementation of an early vascular access assessment program.

Outcomes that should be measured relate to complication rates, dwell time, insertion success rate, and productivity. One outcome that is rarely measured is early assessment. How many VADs did the patient get for their therapy? Did the patient get the right device on day 1 or within 3 days of therapy? Were there preventable complications if the right device had been chosen at the onset of therapy? The measurement of vascular access assessment is not currently being performed in institutions. The traditional measurements related to insertion success and complications have been the primary end points. Future endeavors should concentrate on what outcomes are we seeking for device selection and is there a process improvement that could be accomplished in this direction. At the Association of Vascular Access (AVA 2013) meeting, a speaker discussed the fact that there is a high rate of PIV complications related to phlebitis, infiltration, and patient pullout. In fact, the statement was that almost 30 % of PIVs failed to go the length of treatment. The conclusion was how one makes a 1-in. PIV accomplishes a longer dwell time. The author wondered how one chooses the best VAD to match the patient's therapy needs as maybe the PIV is not the right device. Future endeavors need to establish a worldwide consensus on how to choose a VAD. Santolim et al. [34] initiated such a process on a smaller level at the Institute of Orthopedics and Traumatology in Brazil. Clinical nursing may choose, with the help of an algorithm and education, between a PIV, PICC, CVC, tunneled line, and port. This assessment process has the complete backing of the physician service. By creating a multidisciplinary decision-making algorithm, which also involved pharmacy, the process is flourishing in this facility. It takes a group or team to make major changes in healthcare, and Arlete Mazzini who was the program champion as a nurse director has challenged the system and became a leader in her facility for nursing autonomy on VAD decision making rather than carrying out the placement of a VAD by medical order alone.

As PICC teams move forward into this decade, the implementation of higher-tech tools in the form of tip location and tip navigation may move the actual PICC line procedure into more outpatient arenas and even into the patient's home without hospitalization. Only time and reimbursement will determine where the future leads. Always follow the money trail and that will provide the direction they say. The success of the PICC line and PICC line team has been a result of providing cost-effective therapy [38] with a low complication device. The emphasis on patient infection reduction will also become a larger focus point worldwide. This focus is likely to lead to the development of PICC teams or vascular access specialty teams worldwide. Teams that will have a vested interest in maintaining low infection rates as shown by Harnage [22], on achieving zero infection for 15 months and now going on 7 years, with over 2,000 PICC lines placed a year.

References

1. Alexander M, Corrigan A et al (2010) Infusion Nurses Society Infusion nursing an evidence – based approach, 3rd edn. Saunders/Elsevier, St. Louis
2. Alexandrou E, Spencer T, Frost SA et al (2010) Establishing a nurse-led central venous catheter insertion service. JAVA 15:21–27
3. Agency for Healthcare Research and Quality (2001) Making health care safer: a critical analysis of patient safety practices. AHRQ United States Evidence Report/Technology Assessment No. 43
4. American Board of Internal Medicine (2013) Internal Medicine policies: eligibility for certification and board policies. www.abim.org/certification/policies/imss/im.aspx. Accessed 14 Oct 2013
5. American College of Emergency Physicians (2008) Policy Statement: Emergency ultrasound guidelines. www.acep.org/content.aspx?id=32878. Accessed 15 Oct 2013
6. Anstett M, Royer TI (2003) the impact of ultrasound on PICC placement. JAVA 8:21–28
7. Barton AJ, Danek G, Johns P et al (1998) Improving patient outcomes through CQI: vascular access planning. J Nurs Care Qual 13:77–85
8. Bass HJG, Bashore TM et al (2013) ACCF/AHA/SCAI 2013 update of clinical competence statement. American College of Cardiology Foundation. www.cardiosource.org/Science-And-Quality/Journal-Scan/2013/05ACCF-AHA-S. Accessed 14 Oct 2013
9. Breschan C, Platzer M, Jost R et al (2011) Consecutive prospective case series of a new method for ultrasound-guided supraclavicular approach to the brachiocephalic vein in children. BJABr J Anaesth 106:732–737
10. Bolton D (2010) Writing a business case for the expansion of service: expanding the IV therapy team from start to finish. J Infect Prev 10:S27–S32
11. Burns D (2005) The Vanderbilt PICC service program, procedural, and patient outcomes success. JVAD 10:1–10

12. Burns T, Lamberth B (2010) Facility wide benefits of radiology vascular access teams. Radiol Manage 32:28–32
13. Business Directory (2013) Definition of team. www.businessdictionary.com/defintions/team. html. Accessed 13 Oct 2013
14. Carroll SS, Lashbrook AL (2011) Bronson Methodist Hospital: reducing central line bloodstream infections in critical care units and beyond. Commonwealth Fund 19:1–14
15. Cavanagh P (2005) Ultrasound training recommendations for medical and surgical specialties second edition. Royal College of Radiologists. www.rcr.ac.uk. Accessed 13 Oct 2013
16. Davis J, Kokotis K (2004) A new perspective for PICC line insertion: cost effectiveness and outcomes associated with an independent PICC service. JAVA 9:93–98
17. Dobson C, Meythaler D, Wong P, Ramirez C (2006) On the scene at Banner Estrella Medical Center, the hospital of the future. Nurs Admin Q 30:228–235
18. Dobson L, Wong DG (2001) Development of a successful PICC insertion program. JVAD 6:31–34
19. Ean R, Kirmse J, Roslien J et al (2006) A nurse-driven peripherally inserted central catheter team exhibits excellence through teamwork. JAVA 11:135–143
20. Domino KB, Bowdle TA, Posner KL et al (2004) Injuries and liability related to central vascular catheters: a closed case analysis. Anesthesiology 100:1411–1418
21. Hadaway L (2010) Development of an infusion alliance. J Infus Nurs 33:278–290
22. Harnage SA (2007) Achieving zero catheter related blood stream infections: 15 months success in a community based medical center. JAVA 12:218–224
23. Hornsby S, Matter K, Beets B et al (2005) Cost loses associated with the "PICC, stick and run team" concept. J Infus Nurs 28:45–53
24. Infusion Nurses Society (2011) Infusion nursing standards of practice. J Infus Nurs 34: S1–S110
25. Kokotis K (2005) Cost containment and infusion services. J Infus Nurs 28:S22–S32
26. Kopman DF (2007) Ultrasound-guided internal jugular access: a proposed standardized approach and implications for training and practice. Chest 132:302–309
27. Merriam-Webster Dictionary (2013) Definition of champion. www.merriam-ebster.com/dictionary/champion. Accessed 15 Oct 2013
28. Meyer BM (2010) Implementing and maintaining an infusion alliance. J Infus Nurs 33: 292–303
29. McMahon DD (2002) Evaluating new technology to improve patient outcomes. J Infus Nurs 25:250–252
30. Moureau N, Lamperti M, Kelly LJ (2013) Evidence-based consensus on the insertion of central venous access devices: definition of minimal requirements for training. Br J Anaesth 110:347–356
31. Petit J, Wycoff MM (2007) Peripherally inserted central catheters. National Association of Neonatal Nurses Guidelines and Practice, 2nd edition. www.NANN.org. Accessed 13 Oct 2013
32. Ramierez C, Malloch K, Agee C (2010) Evaluation of respiratory care practitioner central venous catheter insertion program. JAVA 15:207–211
33. Rivera AM, Strauss KW, Van Zundert A et al (2005) The history of peripheral intravenous catheters: how little plastic tubes revolutionized medicine. AcTa Anaseth Belg 56:271–282
34. Santolim TQ, Santos LAU, Mazzini A et al (2012) The strategic role of the nurse in the selection of IV devices. Br J Nurs 21:S28–S32
35. Santolucito JB (2001) A retrospective evaluation of the timeliness of physician initiated PICC referrals. JVAD 6:20–26
36. Sznajder JI, Zveibil FR, Bitterman H et al (1986) Central vein catheterization: failure and complication rates by three percutaneous approaches. Arch Intern Med 146:259–261
37. Terry J, Baranowski L, Lonsway RA et al (1995) Intravenous therapy clinical principles and practice. WB Saunders, St. Louis
38. Todd J (1999) Peripherally inserted central catheters and their use in IV therapy. Br J Nutr 8:140–148

CPSIA information can be obtained
at www.ICGtesting.com
Printed in the USA
LVOW02*0006180416
484014LV00001B/48/P